SUBPRIME HEALTH

Subprime Health

DEBT AND RACE IN U.S. MEDICINE

Nadine Ehlers and Leslie R. Hinkson, Editors

University of Minnesota Press
Minneapolis
London

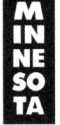

An earlier version of chapter 6 was published as "Race for Cures: Rethinking the Racial Logics of 'Trust' in Biomedicine," *Sociology Compass* 8 (2014): 755–69, http://dx.doi.org/10.1111/soc4.12167. Copyright 2014 John Wiley and Sons Ltd. Reprinted with permission.

Copyright 2017 by the Regents of the University of Minnesota

All rights reserved. No part of this publication may be reproduced, stored in a retrieval system, or transmitted, in any form or by any means, electronic, mechanical, photocopying, recording, or otherwise, without the prior written permission of the publisher.

Published by the University of Minnesota Press
111 Third Avenue South, Suite 290
Minneapolis, MN 55401-2520
http://www.upress.umn.edu

The University of Minnesota is an equal-opportunity educator and employer.

Library of Congress Cataloging-in-Publication Data
Names: Ehlers, Nadine, editor. | Hinkson, Leslie R., editor.
Title: Subprime health : debt and race in U.S. medicine / Nadine Ehlers and Leslie R. Hinkson, editors.
Description: Minneapolis, MN : University of Minnesota Press, [2017] | Includes bibliographical references and index.
Identifiers: LCCN 2016036914 (print) | ISBN 978-1-5179-0149-3 (hc) | ISBN 978-1-5179-0150-9 (pb)
Subjects: | MESH: Health Services Accessibility—economics | African Americans | Cost of Illness | Healthcare Disparities—economics | Racism | United States
Classification: LCC RA448.5.N4 (print) | NLM WA 300 AA1 | DDC 362.1089/96073—dc23
LC record available at https://lccn.loc.gov/2016036914

CONTENTS

Introduction: Race-based Medicine and the Specter of Debt   vii
Nadine Ehlers and Leslie R. Hinkson

PART I. RACE-BASED MEDICINE AND MONETARY DEBT

1 The High Cost of Having Hypertension while   3
  Black in America
  Leslie R. Hinkson

2 "When Treating Patients like Criminals Makes Sense":   31
  Medical Hot Spotting, Race, and Debt
  Nadine Ehlers and Shiloh Krupar

3 Obamacare and Sovereign Debt: Race, Reparations,   55
  and the Haunting of Premature Death
  Jenna M. Loyd

4 BiDil's Compensation Relations   83
  Anne Pollock

PART II. RACE-BASED MEDICINE AND INDEBTEDNESS

5 The Meaning of Health Disparities   107
  Catherine Bliss

6 What Do We Owe Each Other? Moral Debts and   129
  Racial Distrust in Experimental Stem Cell Science
  Ruha Benjamin and Leslie R. Hinkson

7	Lessons from Racial Medicine: The Group, the Individual, and the Equal Protection Clause Khiara M. Bridges	155
	Conclusion: Freedom from Debt? Leslie R. Hinkson and Nadine Ehlers	183
	Acknowledgments	197
	Contributors	199
	Index	201

INTRODUCTION

Race-based Medicine and the Specter of Debt

NADINE EHLERS AND LESLIE R. HINKSON

> Racial inequality is still the unsolved American dilemma. The nation's character has been forged on the contradiction of the promise of equality and its systematic denial. For most of our nation's history we have allowed racial inequality to fester. But there are other choices.
> —MELVIN L. OLIVER AND THOMAS M. SHAPIRO,
> *Black Wealth/White Wealth* (2006)

> Of all the forms of inequality, injustice in health care is the most shocking and inhumane.
> —MARTIN LUTHER KING JR., "A CIVIL RIGHTS ICON'S THOUGHTS ON HEALTH CARE" (1966)

If at the turn of the twentieth century the nation's most pressing problem was that of the color line, by the turn of the twenty-first, many Americans had reason to believe that line was finally disappearing. During that roughly hundred-year period, African Americans would make unprecedented gains in income, educational attainment, and occupational status largely due to the hard-fought struggles of the civil rights era. The end of Jim Crow seemed synonymous with the end of racism in the United States. As if to confirm that the color line was a thing of the past, the nation elected its first African American president in 2008 and then reelected him in 2012. What further proof was needed to demonstrate that race was no longer a significant determinant of one's life chances, of one's access to opportunity?

Evidence clearly suggests that reports of the death of racial inequality in America are both premature and greatly exaggerated. Despite a substantial increase in the share of African Americans joining the middle class from the 1970s until the 1990s, that growth has been stagnant for the past thirty years, and there is some evidence that this number is on the decline. The earnings of Black men are approximately 25 percent lower than those of comparable White men, and employment rates of Black men continue to lag behind those of their White counterparts. In fact, the Black unemployment rate has been twice as high as that for Whites for the past fifty years; nor, in that same amount of time, has the gap in household income between Blacks and Whites narrowed.[1] The wealth gap that exists between Black and White America is astounding: as of 2009, the median White–Black wealth ratio was 19 to 1.[2] Beyond the wealth gap, Black women are three times more likely to be incarcerated than White women, while Black men are six times more likely to be incarcerated than White men.[3] Also as of 2009, 31 percent of Latino households had zero or negative net worth compared to 15 percent of white households, and 27 percent of American Indian and Alaskan Native families with children lived in poverty (and 32 percent of those with children younger than five years). These rates are more than double those of the general population and are even higher in certain tribal communities (66 percent).[4]

One of the clearest indicators of these gaps appears in the health disparities by race that haunt the American health care system. From its inception, this system has racialized both access to and quality of care. In our present moment, Blacks continue to experience a higher incidence of hypertension, diabetes, colorectal cancer, infant mortality, and HIV infection rates than any other racial or ethnic group in the country—to name just a few of the race gaps in morbidity rates that exist today. One might offer the pithy observation that Blacks continue to enjoy a lot less of the good stuff and a lot more of the bad despite the many strides in racial progress the United States has witnessed over the past century. Health disparities are also found among other racial and ethnic minorities. Latinos, as a whole, experience higher rates of diabetes, HIV infection, tuberculosis, cervical cancer, stomach cancer, liver cancer, and liver disease than Whites.[5] These numbers are even starker when we disaggregate by country of origin, as some subgroups within the Latino population experience even higher morbidity and mortality rates associated with these and several other diseases. In Native American and Alaskan adults, the age-adjusted death rate far exceeds the general population, by almost 40 percent, and deaths due to chronic liver disease and cirrhosis, tuberculosis, pneumonia, influenza, and heart disease also exceed those of the general population.[6] Although often left out of the discussion, health disparities also exist within the Asian American and Pacific Islander communities. For example, Asian Americans experience the highest rates of any racial or ethnic group for liver, uterine, cervical, and stomach cancer.[7] Asian Americans and Pacific Islanders have greater incidence rates of tuberculosis and hepatitis B than any other racial or ethnic group, and Asian Americans experience higher rates of diabetes than Whites.[8]

Many see race-based medicine as a key way to address the persistence of racial inequalities in health. Targeting health care and medical intervention according to race can broadly be viewed as a way to pay back the debt that is owed to minorities for past and ongoing medical mistreatment, undertreatment, neglect, or disenfranchisement in relation to attaining health. Such attention to race as it intersects with medicine is generally seen as a good. Social analysts, however, often tell a different story, questioning the scientific, financial, and moral integrity of this practice and suggesting instead that race-based medicine creates new debts and compounds old ones. The essays in this volume seek to intervene into the discussion around race-based medicine by looking at its relationship with debt. If race-based medicine is increasingly supplanting attention to structural factors as the means through which to attend to deeply entrenched health inequalities, what are the unintended consequences? Indeed, what are the costs of race-based medicine itself?

Throughout this volume, we foreground the ways race-based medicine intersects with the concept of debt in myriad ways and across multiple contexts. What ties race-based medicine and debt together is the health debt that has accumulated throughout the African American community over the course of four centuries. This debt relates to the foregone health and medical resources that could have been invested in minority communities in the past but were not due to racism, segregation, and even benign neglect. It relates to the disproportionate disease burden that minorities carry as a result of these past practices, creating bodies of dependency. It relates to the monetary debt that minority communities and society as a whole accumulate as health care costs are on the rise and continue to be unregulated while programs designed to help ameliorate health disparities lose funding across the country. And it relates to the corporeal, financial, and psychological costs that minorities have had to bear as a consequence of their otherness. Race-based medicine thus operates in and through a web of debt and indebtedness.

Mapping the Terrain of Race-based Medicine

As the cost of health care grows in the United States, individuals and entire communities are increasingly faced with the crushing debt that often accompanies such growth. Racial and ethnic minorities are particularly vulnerable to the negative effects of the rising cost of health care. Many have lower rates of health insurance coverage, have lower levels of income and wealth to pay for medical services out of pocket, and are less able to access affordable care. This negatively affects their economic health and exerts a negative impact on their physical health. For example, uninsured people are less likely to receive recommended care for disease prevention and management, often resulting in an increase in the incidence and severity of a number of diseases. These factors are evidenced both in the 2010 census, which reported that 20.8 percent of Blacks and 30.7 percent of Latinos had no insurance coverage compared to 11.7 percent of Whites,[9] and in the U.S. Department of Health and Human Services 2013 *National Healthcare Quality Report,* which found that minorities lack adequate cancer screening, dental care, counseling about diet and exercise, and flu vaccination in addition to receiving poor management for diseases such as diabetes.[10] Overall, the U.S. Department of Health and Human Services has determined that "health care quality and access are suboptimal, especially for minority and low-income groups," such that while "quality [of health care] is improving, access and disparities are not."[11]

Lower rates of insured status among Blacks and other minorities, compounded by inequities in the quality of and overall access to care received, are all symptomatic of a health care system that has yet to shed its racialized past. But the rising cost of health care has also arguably stratified care more sharply along class lines over the past few decades. Given that race and wealth are so closely correlated in the United States, this portends an even stronger link between economic and physical health, a fact that is particularly stark in Black communities.[12] Less wealth understandably leads many to forego medical care, and it unilaterally constrains the ability to achieve and maintain health. Wealth inequality then contributes to health inequality in the United States. Health inequality in turn compounds wealth inequality, as lower rates of health insurance coverage and limited health care options put certain racial and ethnic groups at greater financial risk. Again, this is especially true for Blacks: when asked about their medical bills and medical debt, 44 percent of Black adults younger than 65 years old reported that they were unable to pay their medical bills or had outstanding medical debt compared to 33 percent of Whites and 29 percent of Latinos. When narrowing the focus to include only uninsured adults younger than 65 years old, 61 percent of Blacks reported having problems paying their medical bills or outstanding medical debt compared to 56 percent of Whites and 35 percent of Latinos.[13] While researchers debate whether the direction of causality is greater wealth leading to better health or vice versa, what becomes evident in tracing the history of the American health care system is an enduring reality of race-based health disparity that is inextricable from wealth inequality and the tyranny of debt.

Racial health disparities are by no means a recent phenomenon. As far back as the late nineteenth century, African American sociologist W. E. B. Du Bois demonstrated in his infamous *The Philadelphia Negro* (1899) that vast cleavages in racialized health have long existed in the United States. Importantly, however, he insisted that disease, health, bodily welfare, and indeed the contours of biological life are not ontological—that is, they cannot be explained as the natural state of the bodies of citizens. Instead, as he showed, race-based health disparities arise from broader economic, environmental, social, and political forms of inequality, and thus problems regarding health are "largely a matter of the *condition* of living"—conditions that can often be traced to the nations' origins in settler colonialism and slavery.[14] It is precisely because of these conditions of living that "not everyone in the United States enjoys the same health opportunities . . . . [and] minority Americans experience poorer than average health outcomes from cradle to the grave."[15]

Contemporary inequity might at least partly be explained as the result of a set of choices made in the United States whereby health care was constructed—and generally continues to exist—as a privatized good, with access largely dependent on wealth, income, or employment status. As Republican senator Robert Taft proclaimed in 1949, "It has always been assumed in this country that those able to pay for medical care would buy their own medical service, just as under any system, except a socialistic system, they buy their own food, their own housing, their own clothing, and their own automobiles."[16] What Taft raised here was an ideology of personal responsibility for medical care—a viewpoint that has been a continuing thread in national policy related to medical health care in the decades since his claim, and a sentiment that is only augmented within the contours of neoliberalism. Personal responsibility characterizes the neoliberal era, which has revived and intensified laissez-faire individualism and which has subjected almost every aspect of life to the logic and imperatives of the market. As a consequence, "disaggregated, anxious individuals . . . [are] left more or less to their own devices in the ruthless (and rigged) global competition for power and material reward, answerable to themselves alone for their success or failures."[17] The aftermath of such a position, as Rosemary A. Stevens has noted, is that "after 60 years of experiment [with health policy and the health care industry], an estimated 47 million Americans are uninsured. Over and above this, an unaccounted number are underinsured for services they might need (and be billed for) any day."[18] Given that access to health care is linked to capital—that is, the capacity to pay for it—everyone either goes into debt or is potentially at risk of going into debt in relation to medical expenditure. This is borne out in findings that in 2008, health care bills were the cause of most personal bankruptcies; as of that year, Americans spent more on health insurance and services than they did on food or housing.[19]

In a circular operation, this set of choices regarding health care feeds into and compounds the history and present of racial inequality formed by the workings of structural racism and practices of neglect, dispossession, and abandonment. Such inequality is evident in a first sense in that minorities have been and continue to be subject to what Henry Giroux calls an unbenign "biopolitics of disposability": operations of power in which entire populations are marginalized by race, and socially and environmentally excluded from general processes that foster the life of the population.[20] This exclusion can clearly be seen in regard to biomedicine in the form of lack of access to care and health insurance and in inequities in caregiving.[21] Beyond the realm of biomedicine, however, minority citizens are subjected to dispossession and abandonment through the dismantling of the social wage (via the destruction of social welfare), through the rising rates of incarceration of Black and Brown men and women, and through various practices (such as attacks on the funding of public education and de facto segregation in schools and communities) that lead or contribute to patterns of cumulative disadvantage.

In a second sense, racial inequality is evident in the ways that African Americans in particular are systematically exposed to what Rinaldo Walcott has called "zones of black death." These are spaces (metaphorical or literal) wherein Blacks are imperiled, where "black subjects continue to be marginalized and, as so many practical human actions reveal, put to death."[22] The biomedical arena is undeniably one such zone in that Black subjects have often been harmed rather than healed by the medical embrace. Examples abound, including J. Marion Sims's gynecological experimentation on the bodies of slave women in the 1800s; the grave robbing of Black corpses for various forms of medical study from the 1800s into the 1900s; the Tuskegee syphilis experiments, which spanned 1932 to 1972; and the disproportionate number of Black men diagnosed with schizophrenia in the 1960s, in large part due to their connection with civil rights protest activities.[23] More broadly, however, many minority citizens exist within zones of death. Racial and ethnic minorities are more likely to live in areas where hazardous waste sites, industrial pollution, and lead exposure are prevalent. Landfills and transfer stations, power plants, incinerators, and major highways are also more commonly situated in communities of color, creating health risks for minority populations.[24] Even though minorities have a higher likelihood of residing in places that result in the need for more access to care, they are perversely also more likely to live in communities where access to care is limited. These examples illustrate that what is commonly referred to as race-based medicine need not be confined to specific medical treatments; it may also encompass a broader structure of health care delivery that has contributed to the neglect, even abuse, of minorities over time.

Despite the persistence of racial inequities, the past three decades have seen an ideological shift from race-conscious to color-blind policies throughout American society.[25] This shift has been evidenced not just in popular opinion but also in the judicial system. In a landmark decision in 2007 *(Parents Involved in Community Schools v. Seattle School District No. 1)*, the U.S. Supreme Court ruled that it was unconstitutional for school districts to use individualized racial classifications to achieve diversity and/or avoid racial isolation through student assignment. In his written remarks in the plurality opinion, Chief Justice Roberts famously remarked, "The way to stop discrimination on the basis of race is to stop discriminating on the basis of race."[26] Thus, minority students who were subject to the consequences of de facto racial segregation in their school districts were not deemed subject to the kind of discrimination that the majority felt constituted a compelling interest. The White students, however, who were in danger of being assigned to certain schools in order to help avoid racial isolation, were deemed subject to such discrimination and thus in need of the court's protection. This case is but one demonstration of how the rhetoric of color-blindness has overtaken the broader social arena, matched by a resounding neoliberal insistence on the existence of a supposed level playing field determined by a neutral market.

Paradoxically, race consciousness is on the uptake in biomedicine, and millions of dollars have been targeted in recent years toward research, development, and marketing of race-based pharmaceuticals and treatments. The mapping of the human genome, as a case in point, seemed to offer not just unlimited opportunities for understanding and curing a host of simple and complex diseases and disorders but also a way for the private sector to reap unprecedented profits through investing in new drug technologies. With the promise of individualized medicine that the mapping of the genome seemed to portend, drug companies would enjoy an ever-expanding market that would focus not just on specific diseases but also on specific body types. One drug might cure or at least treat heart disease in a body like yours, while another would cure or treat heart disease in a body like your spouse's or like your neighbor's. Through pursuing a research and marketing strategy that rested on the hypothesis that the same disease actually worked differently in different bodies—or were indeed totally different diseases in different bodies—the pharmaceutical industry and its many investors realized a strategy that would result in not simply the expansion of the creation and supply of targeted treatments but also an incredible rise in the demand for such drugs. There already exist hair care products targeted specifically for blondes, brunettes, or redheads; why not a treatment for skin cancer that does the same? Biomedical researchers, stating up front that race is not a biological category but then claiming it is the best approximation we have for understanding as yet undiscovered genetic markers for race, increasingly turned their attention to developing drugs that targeted specific racial groups.

Two things should be noted about the justifications often cited for increased investment in pharmaceutical development and the expansion of the field of ethnopharmacogenomics. First, there is an assumption that investigating a specific type of "groupness" will lead to better, more individualized, and targeted cures. Indeed, this may be the case when there are scientific reasons for believing the group in question shares specific genetic markers that truly make them a group apart. For example, developing a treatment that targets individuals who are missing a specific enzyme for metabolizing certain drugs or proteins focuses on a group known to share specific genetic markers that may require tailored pharmaceutical interventions. However, scientific researchers do not always use sound theoretical reasons for grouping people. As a case in point, multiple studies have shown the association between astrological sign and health.[27] Does the statistical association found in such studies merit the serious consideration of creating different drugs for a Pisces than an Aries? Does racial grouping operate more like the former example of groupness, or the latter? Second, the expansion of ethnopharmacogenomics is often justified on the basis of its supposed capacity to help ameliorate health disparities and to widen pharmaceutical markets (to those not previously reached and attended to), and by these means pay back a debt for past mistreatment, abuse, or neglect in medicine. Again, race-based medicine—in this case in the form of ethnopharmacogenomics—is linked to the concept of debt.[28]

For the purposes of our focus in this volume, we understand debt, in its broadest sense, as referring to money, goods, and services owing, and indebtedness as referring to being in a state of dependency or under an obligation to pay or return something. Debt can be viewed as something owed a group: a history of racialized dispossession, medical neglect, and overexposure to biomedical harms or biomedicalized forms of governance has accumulated a debt to certain racial groups. This debt inversely constructs a state of indebtedness—that is, a duty to attempt to redress past and enduring racial harm. Importantly, we might see this debt as a matter of reparations, what Robert Westley identifies as "compensation to victims of injustice . . . or even remorse in the form of public acknowledgement of wrongdoing."[29] Although these histories—produced through settler colonialism, slavery, and racialized segregation or discrimination—can never be undone and the debt never fully defrayed, adopting a framework of reparations ideally "affirms and reconfigures the past as a vehicle for social change."[30] As Stephen Best and Saidiya Hartman have noted, "Assessing debt and calculating injury [may] itself [be] a formula for justice."[31] In addition to being what is owed a group, then, debt can be what a group carries—in this case, white societal debt to minorities.

Is it possible for race-based medicine to refigure the past and pave the way forward toward resolution of debts owed? Can it be a form of affirmation of past wrongs and reparation of the state of indebtedness? Or do we see a promise that remains frustrated wherein race-based medicine actually perpetuates injustice and compounds the arching history of debt? We would hazard that race-based medicine cannot be viewed in binary terms—debt able to be paid versus further debt accrued—because this is too simple a characterization. Instead, certain forms of racial targeting in biomedicine might offer a form of reparations that Alyosha Goldstein identifies as "recompense aimed at securing business as usual."[32] Also, certain forms of race-based medicine can be said to perversely shift the responsibility of paying the debt of past injustice to the racially disadvantaged individual or community: failing to alter material conditions and instead obligating minorities to become responsible for their own health, to access supposedly appropriate treatment, and to take on racial difference as a presocial or extrasocial truth. There is nothing new in the maneuver of shifting responsibility of debt to the disadvantaged. As Hartman has powerfully argued, African Americans have historically been constructed as indebted to society and the nation: "The very bestowal of freedom established the indebtedness of the freed through a calculus of blame and responsibility that mandated that the formerly enslaved both repay this investment of faith and prove their worthiness."[33] Such payment was to be made through Blacks showing they were able to take on the onus of accountability, self-reliance, and self-responsibility—the traits associated with liberal individuality—in the face of slavery and its aftermath, and with an absence of resources to do so. White responsibility for centuries of subjugation was evacuated; instead, "the bound and sovereign self of rights was . . . answerable to his failures; social relations thereby receded before the singular exercise of the will and the blameworthy and isolated individual."[34] While the burden of self-responsibility inevitably extends to all, it is important to heed Goldstein's claim (particularly pronounced in the neoliberal era) that for minorities, "the affirmation of the self-owning individual reinvigorates rather than challenges the terms of dispossession."[35]

Race-based medicine, as the contributions to this volume insist, is inextricable from the logics and operations of debt because it involves the creation of debt or debts, of debtors and creditors, and of states of owing that remain unpaid and passed on. For example, while one of the motivations for pursuing the development of race-based pharmaceuticals might be to help eliminate health disparities, the millions of dollars devoted to such pursuits can also be seen as sucking away resources that could go toward immediately reducing health disparities in ways that have been proven to be effective, thus maintaining the health debt that exists in many minority communities. In another example, when an individual does not have access to affordable care as a result of broader operations of racial inequality, every time she goes to the doctor, she runs the risk of incurring debt.[36] As a case in point, Blacks and Latinos are more likely to access care from the emergency department for conditions that could be treated by a primary care physician at lower expense. However, given that they have fewer alternatives for accessing care after regular working hours or on the weekends than other groups—primarily a function of geography and type of medical coverage—they resort to accessing emergency care that can cost upward of twenty times what it would cost at a clinic or private practice. The connection between debt and race-based medicine is also evident in the fact that many hospitals located in or

INTRODUCTION   xvii

near communities of color have had to close their doors because of uncompensated health care debt, which is generated when people in their communities are unable to pay their health care bills.[37] These closures often result in less access to care for the people who once relied on their services, higher unemployment in those communities (the result of job losses from the closures), and less favorable health outcomes. Ultimately these various permutations of debt need to be recognized in order to appreciate the nuances of race-based medicine and its stakes.

To facilitate exploration of the debt logics that surface within and subtend race-based medicine, we offer three key definitions of what we understand as race-based medicine. First, race-based medicine can be defined as the systematic targeting of racial groups for special consideration when diagnosing certain ailments or treating certain diseases. This targeting is based on information as varied as purported differences in biological responses to specific treatments; purported behavioral differences across groups vis-à-vis biomedicine and biomedical treatment; purported differences in the health literacy of certain groups; and the purported correlation between the value certain individuals place on their own lives and the lives of others like them and their racial group affiliation. Race-based medicine, operating through this form of targeting, encompasses practices in clinical encounters, treatment, and diagnosis. This way of understanding race-based medicine, however, leads into our second definition, for, as Sharona Hoffman has noted, "As this approach develops, physicians may prescribe different dosages of medication for people of separate 'races' or may provide them with entirely different drugs."[38] Thus, following from our first definition, race-based medicine can also be understood as race-targeted pharmaceutical interventions for specific diseases. Under this definition, race-based medicine can extend to the whole field of ethnopharmacogenomics, which uses race and ethnicity as proxies for specific genotypes or phenotypes that are thought to be associated with differential disease risk and drug response. This is perhaps the narrowest definition of race-based medicine, and it is exemplified in the well-known case of BiDil, a heart failure therapy that was the first U.S. Food and Drug Administration (FDA)-approved pharmaceutical with a racial indication.[39] Many critics echo Dorothy Roberts's contention that race-based medicine, when it is understood in this sense, is scientifically flawed, commercially motivated, and politically dangerous.[40] Third, and operating at a more macro level, race-based medicine can be defined as an entire system of health and medical care delivery that uses race as a primary means of rationing and rationalizing care. This is our broadest definition, and it takes into account the differentiation of bodies within biomedicine, the question of who gets access to health coverage, what types of care are available, and how many doctors or what kinds of care are available in particular communities. Understood in these terms, race-based medicine would encapsulate historical and contemporary segregation (both de jure and de facto) in health care, where individuals have been and continue to be treated by separate doctors and in separate hospitals according to race.[41] This is our preferred definition of race-based medicine, as it encapsulates both the two previous meanings as well as the pervasive nature of race-driven thinking that informs biomedical practices and health care delivery in the United States.

It is important to note that alternative understandings of race itself are often at work within race-based medicine. On the one hand, race is often framed in essentialist terms as a fixed biological reality: as "the product of evolutionary processes acting on (more or less) genetically isolated populations."[42] Such a view has not only recently resurfaced in the scientific community (in relation to a determinedly race-focused genomics) but is also gaining currency in the public domain, with direct consumer use of DNA tests to discover genetic ancestry and the emergence of ethnopharmacogenomics.[43] On the other hand, race is also framed in nonessentialist terms in race-based medicine. Here, while race groupings or categories are not seen to reflect innate human biological variation, they are viewed as tools (although they may be inaccurate or inadequate for understanding genetic diversity). With this approach, race is often used as a proxy for communities and disease groups, becoming what might be seen as a label of convenience.[44] Even if race is understood as social rather than innate within this framework, in practice, it is invariably reduced to or reified as a biological reality.

In this volume, we view race as a set of meanings that have been assigned to the body. These meanings are historically and culturally specific and shift over time. In chorus with many critical race scholars in the humanities and social sciences, we maintain that the meanings that are ascribed to particular bodies—bodies that are named as racially distinct, based most generally on phenotype—are the invention of cultural practices and social institutions and operate as ways to demarcate and stratify that difference.[45] Racial meanings, however, also register at the level of the body. This can be understood in two key ways. First, despite being a social concept and precisely because it is a political category, race maps out material existence: it influences such things as health, education, housing, employment options, and interpersonal relationships; further, race conditions the ways that individuals live through the body. In this sense, as Ian Haney López has argued, "race is neither an essence nor an illusion."[46] Because racial meanings and their effects are consistently reinforced, challenged, reworked, and revised in the social arena, race itself must be seen as "an ongoing, contradictory, self-reinforcing, plastic process subject to macro forces of social and political struggle and the micro effects of daily decisions."[47] Second, because racial meanings map out material existence, race has biological effects. By this we mean that the differentiation of bodies—based on supposed innate racial particularity—and the accumulative effect of racial discrimination based on this differentiation condition the biological life of an individual. Troy Duster perhaps marks this relationship most succinctly when he refutes the supposed correlation between Blackness and the propensity to develop hypertension: "If you follow me around Nordstrom, and put me in jail at nine times the rate of whites, and refuse to give me a bank loan, I might get hypertensive. What's generating my increased blood pressure are the social forces at play, not my DNA." Stressing the point, he argues that the issue of heart failure in Blacks "was not biological or genetic in origin, but biological in effect due to stress-related outcomes of reduced access to valued social goods, such as employment, promotion, and housing stock. The effect was biological, not the origins."[48]

As a concept, however, race has been deployed since the eighteenth century, when naturalists used it to organize human diversity. As Kelly Happe has noted, race is then both a scientific concept and a "rhetorical artefact":

> As a scientific concept, it organizes and condenses the materiality
> of the object world: in this case, the materiality of human diversity.
> As a rhetorical term, it is a partial snapshot of complex patterns
> of human evolutionary history, rendering certain aspects of human
> diversity prominent (for instance, "primary" continent of origin) and
> thus meaningful, rendering other aspects of human diversity (such as
> admixture) insignificant.[49]

Happe's critique points to the reality that basing medical care and treatment on race has become an increasingly thorny issue in the scientific, biomedical, and social arenas. While much of the debate over race-based medicine has been centered around its effectiveness or even its appropriateness (if race is not a biological reality, why use it as such in the medical encounter? Is this "good" or "bad" medicine?), one key benefit to viewing race-based medicine through the lens of debt is that it brings into focus the moral, ethical, and even efficiency debates surrounding the issue, and importantly, it compels us to move beyond thinking about race-based medicine within a specifically bioscientific/biomedical framework to instead think about it as a sociopolitical phenomenon. As such, race-based medicine is driven by several key motivations, which tend to fall under the following four broad categories:

1. Benevolence—Race-based medicine is a reparative means of addressing historical wrongs that may have led to contemporary health disparities.
2. Self-interest—Race-based medicine is a means of making a profit while also fulfilling a public need (here, capital accumulation might be understood as a form of neoimperialism).
3. Upholding scientific "truth"—Among "true believers," race is a biological reality, and although past research indicates otherwise, it is in the interest of science that race-based medicine be practiced, studied, and justified.
4. Reducing government spending—As the cost of health care continues to grow as a share of both public and private expenditures, racially targeted approaches to the delivery of health care—particularly in low-income communities—are introduced as a means of reducing the government portion of its cost.[50]

Additionally, these motivations lead to a wide range of costs that create a system of debtors and creditors. While we have touched on some of these already, these costs might include the following:

1. The cost of funding race-based biomedical research that to date has yielded little to no benefit, often at the expense of other programs and projects that have been proven to effectively reduce health disparities.
2. The negative costs that race-based medicine/medical practices often have on the social life and dignity of minority subjects.
3. The reentrenchment of social divisions and the securing of notions of racial ontology that can result from race-based medicine/medical practices.
4. The possibility of improper diagnoses and treatments that can create added burdens for individuals, communities, and health systems in terms of the cost of care, limitations on individual earnings due to diminished health, and elevated mortality and morbidity rates that affect the overall health, vitality, and wealth of communities over time.

A second benefit derived from examining race-based medicine through the lens of debt is that it compels a consideration of larger scales of operation: through the lens of debt, the discussion moves beyond the almost myopic focus on genes and genomics that much of the current literature on race-based medicine has adopted and allows us to extend our analysis to include whole individuals, neighborhoods and communities, and larger-scale systems of governance. Ultimately, we see that race-based medicine and its implications occupy a fraught terrain, particularly in terms of how it is linked to debt.

To explore these ideas, we have organized the book into two sections that reflect key themes of debt that our contributors believe are often neglected in current debates surrounding race-based medicine. These themes bring together both the primary motivations that drive race-based medicine and the costs associated with a system of medical care, treatment, and research that encourages the use of race as a central organizing principle.

The first part addresses issues of monetary debt associated with race-based medicine. The contributors illustrate how monetary debt associated with race-based medicine disproportionately burdens individuals and entire communities, and how monetary debt and race are implicated in and conditioned by broader relations of power. Given our earlier discussion of the wealth gap that exists between Whites and minorities in the United States, the issue of disproportionate debt load associated with race-based medicine clearly extends beyond the medical realm.

Leslie Hinkson focuses on monetary debts that individuals accrue that are due to race-based patterns of pharmaceutical prescription. Specifically, she finds that Black women, although more likely to be unmarried and uninsured, as well as more likely to experience higher levels of poverty than other groups, are disproportionately prescribed more expensive drug treatments for hypertension than their White and male counterparts. Not only does this pattern of prescription illustrate the ways that race-targeted recommendations for pharmacological interventions follow a logic independent of established guidelines for suitable care but it also shows how this logic works to increase the financial vulnerability of an already vulnerable group. Nadine Ehlers and Shiloh Krupar explore the recent phenomenon of race-targeted medical hot spotting. This practice, as they explain, identifies "high utilizers" of the health system (using medical data collection, Geographic Information Systems, and the principles of spatialized racial profiling) in order to minimize the uncompensated health care debt carried by hospitals that treat uninsured patients. They focus on how attempts to lower the monetary debt incurred by hospitals—through this new form of race-based medicine—situates minorities as responsible for this debt and actually reentrenches racial disparity. Jenna M. Loyd's chapter discusses how the partisan battle over the Affordable Care Act sheds light on the ways race and identity politics have been "always present and made absent" in political debates over sovereign debt and medicine. Specifically, she shows how the framing of the congressional debate over the passage of the Affordable Care Act carefully papered over all discussion of race such that the relationship between universal health care and the past and present harms of structural racism was all but erased from public discourse—except in the hands of conservative commentators who decried any attempts to address historical wrongs as unjust and unwarranted. While focused on the U.S. health care system and the ways it has effectively rationed access to care along racial lines, this chapter more broadly addresses how public policy has historically been crafted to exclude and isolate African Americans from the prerequisites of full citizenship—exclusions that demand some form of reparative justice that the nation's cultural and political bent toward color-blindness will never admit or allow. In the final chapter in this section, Anne Pollock asks who pays the cost—that is, who carries the debt for race-based medicine? She looks to the marketing (and market failure) of the race-specific pharmaceutical, BiDil, and what she calls the drugs' accompanying compensation relations. For Pollock, this is "a concept that seeks to track not only debt ledgers but also the lines of value transfers—that is, relations between the pharmaceutical company and the physicians that performed the trial on the one hand, and the U.S. Food and Drug Administration (FDA) that approved its race-based indication on the other; and between the pharmaceutical company and patients as mediated through the complex array of public and private payers." Looking to compensation relations, as highlighted in Pollock's account, allows us to view racialized medicine not through the lens of what is owed but through the lens of what is given—financially and otherwise—and how this is always affected by broader relations of power in a racially stratified society. This chapter ultimately situates costs associated with race-based drugs within the broader political economy of race-based medicine and shows how these are linked to monetary debt.

The second part focuses on the relationships between indebtedness and race-based medicine. As marked out earlier, we conceptualize indebtedness as states of owing and/or dependency. Indebtedness might illustrate the relationship between race-based medicine and states of dependency as well as moral debt. Regarding dependency, indebtedness refers to a citizenship status that constructs one's identity as being perpetually in debt to and dependent on the state. Moral debt might here be imagined as the debt that the medical establishment—and society at large—owes for the past and present neglect and abuses of many communities of color. This debt is a moral one precisely because it is concerned with the principles of just action and the ethical question of how we want to live as a society. While race-based medicine might at times be viewed as a mechanism of reparative justice, moral debts can also be accrued through race-based medicine, in its inability to meet the clinical obligation to "do no harm."

Our first contributor in this section, Catherine Bliss, examines the ways that the institutionalization of the sociogenomic paradigm has created perverse incentives for social science researchers to shift their focus from the social determinants of health and health disparities to a more genome-focused one. In an environment where "all publicly funded research is beholden to the racial impetus," not only has research in health disparities grown more dependent on funding that minimizes structural conditions (which largely explain racial gaps in rates of morbidity and mortality) but also the process of knowledge production in the field is compromised by the state of dependency researchers find themselves in when pursuing funding opportunities. Ruha Benjamin and Leslie R. Hinkson investigate how biomedical trial recruitment discourse constructs racial group boundaries that potentially undermine not only the level of trust research subjects must place in researchers but also the attempts of researchers to use science and medicine to redress prior forms of abuse and neglect, particularly of African Americans. Through framing trust as a cultural trait that some racial groups have more or less of than others, researchers effectively ignore the larger institutionalized structures of inequality in biomedicine and beyond that shape relationships of trust. It also blinds them to how they themselves contribute to present-day levels of distrust of medicine and biomedical research within certain communities of color and the harm that this inflicts on these communities. Broadly speaking, this chapter illustrates how reparative justice schemes are often undermined by both the relatively ahistorical framing of these plans and the often racialized lens through which researchers and practitioners view their subjects and patients in the first place. Concluding this section, Khiara M. Bridges offers a comparison of the U.S. Supreme Court's arguments regarding the use of race in college admissions with that found in the field of biomedicine, and the potential crossovers and problematics that such a comparison reveals. While the core of the initial impetus for enacting affirmative action legislation was repaying debts to marginalized communities for past societal wrongs, since the 1980s, the Supreme Court has worked to dismantle this function. With biomedicine, however, the use of race has been defended as a vehicle for addressing decades of abuse and neglect characterizing much of its past relationship to communities of color. At the core of her argument is whether the use of race in one area is individuating or not and whether this distinction holds the key to devising policies to address issues of reparative justice that will withhold legal challenges. As her analysis reveals, both biomedicine and the law are flawed in their understanding of what race is and how it operates. Contrary to the Supreme Court's majority decision on affirmative action and its uses, race can be individuating as part of a college admissions file in that it places the life of the individual in specific context. And contrary to the logics of biomedicine, race cannot be individuating in that it obscures the genetic profile of individuals by grouping them into imaginary biological categories that are in fact very real political ones. Her work ultimately provides a theoretical frame for understanding the ways race does and does not work to offer real insights about individuals. In the conclusion of the volume, we trace the primary thematics that tie these offerings together and the possible ways forward for rethinking race and race-based medicine.

We note that many of the following chapters focus on the case of Blacks in general and African Americans in particular. As we have illustrated throughout this introduction, race-based medicine is not something that affects only African Americans. However, the Black–White difference has historically framed the issue, and African Americans today are the primary targets of race-based medical strategies. We hope this volume encourages subsequent work that sheds more light on the ways that race-based medicine affects the health, lives, and life chances of other groups both within and beyond the geographical boundaries of the United States. We believe the volume offers a bridge between more positivistic investigations of medicine and its association with health disparities and more theoretical, critical approaches to the same. It speaks just as directly to the social determinants of health, the critical race, and the anthropology and sociology of medicine literatures. Indeed, we believe that our contributions vividly illustrate various ways biomedicine itself contributes to racial disparities—as opposed to mere differences—in health outcomes.

Taken together, the following chapters illustrate that debt is central to race-based medicine. These essays show that the focus on race in medicine and the hard sciences creates unintended consequences—forms of debt. Not only does race-based medicine lead to the disproportionate accumulation of monetary debt to certain communities but it also works to undermine the ethical obligations that medical practitioners and providers have to the communities they serve. Additionally, race-based medicine perversely attempts to rectify a past debt that was often produced through biomedical knowledge, research, and practice in the first place. We hope that these explorations challenge readers to think through uncomfortable questions that are not often asked in conjunction with race-based medicine. Ultimately, such difficult considerations are necessary if we are to attend to the persistent injustices that structure life in the United States.

Notes

1. Algernon Austin, "The Unfinished March: An Overview," *Economic Policy Institute*, June 18, 2013, http://www.epi.org/.

2. Paul Taylor, Rakesh Kochhar, Richard Fry, Gabriel Velasco, and Seth Motel, *Wealth Gaps Rise to Record Highs between Whites, Blacks, and Hispanics* (Washington, D.C.: Pew Research Center Social and Demographic Trends, 2011), http://www.pewsocialtrends.org/files/2011/07/SDT-Wealth-Report_7-26-11_FINAL.pdf.

3. "King's Dream Remains an Elusive Goal: Many Americans See Racial Disparities," *Pew Research Center Social and Demographic Trends*, August 22, 2013, http://www.pewsocialtrends.org/.

4. On American Indian and Native Alaskan statistics, see Michelle Sarche and Paul Spicer, "Poverty and Health Disparities for American Indian and Alaska Native Children: Current Knowledge and Future Prospects," *Annals of the New York Academy of Sciences* 1136 (2008): 126–36.

5. William A. Vega, Michael A. Rodriguez, and Elisabeth Gruskin, "Health Disparities in the Latino Population," *Epidemiologic Reviews* 31, no. 1 (2009): 99–112.

6. See Sarche and Spicer, "Poverty and Health Disparities."

7. Moon S. Chen Jr., "Cancer Health Disparities among Asian Americans: What We Do and What We Need to Do," *Cancer* 104 (12 suppl) (2005): 2895–902.

8. See Chandak Ghosh, "Healthy People 2010 and Asian Americans/Pacific Islanders: Defining a Baseline of Information," *American Journal of Public Health* 93, no. 12 (2003): 2093–98; and Marguerite J. McNeely and Edward J. Boyko, "Type 2 Diabetes Prevalence in Asian Americans: Results of a National Health Survey," *Diabetes Care* 27, no. 1 (2004): 66–69.

9. Carmen DeNavas-Walt, Bernadette D. Proctor, and Jessica C. Smith, *Income, Poverty, and Health Insurance Coverage in the United States, 2011* (Washington, D.C.: U.S. Department of Commerce, Economics and Statistics Administration, U.S. Census Bureau, 2012), Current Population Report P60-243.

10. Agency for Healthcare Research and Quality (AHRQ), U.S. Department of Health and Human Services, "National Healthcare Disparities Report, 2013: Chapter 10—Access to Health Care," http://www.ahrq.gov/.

11. AHRQ, U.S. Department of Health and Human Services, "Disparities in Healthcare Quality among Racial and Ethnic Minority Groups: Selected Findings from the 2010 National Healthcare Quality and Disparities Report," Fact Sheet, Publication 11-0005-3-EF, http://www.ahrq.gov/. For instance, Blacks are more likely to report using the emergency department for conditions that could have been treated by a primary care physician if one had been available, regardless of whether they had health insurance. This may be attributed to a combination of Blacks on average having more health problems and fewer options for accessing alternative sources of health care after hours and on weekends than their White counterparts. See Commonwealth Fund, "African Americans Have the Highest Rates of Medical Bills and Medical Debt" (New York: Commonwealth Fund, 2005), an interactive chart, from the Commonwealth Fund Biennial Health Insurance Survey, at http://www.commonwealthfund.org/~/media/files/publications/issue-brief/2006/aug/health-care-disconnect--gaps-in-coverage-and-care-for-minority-adults--findings-from-the-commonwealt/doty_issue_brief_figures_not_used_in_quark_but_fin-pdf.pdf.

12. In 2009, the median net worth or wealth of White households was $113,149 while that of Black households was merely $5,667. These figures reflect a decline in inflation-adjusted median wealth of 16 percent for Whites and 53 percent for Blacks from 2005 levels and reveal not only the existence of a significant racial wealth gap between Whites and Blacks but that the latter group's assets were more vulnerable to the effects of the bursting housing bubble in 2006 and ensuing recession from 2007 to 2009. On these figures of decline, see Taylor et al., *Wealth Gaps Rise*. In 2010, White families had on average over six times the wealth of Black families. In real dollar terms, this translates into $632,000 versus $98,000, respectively. In the same year, less than half of Black families owned their own homes, compared to three-quarters of White families. This gap in rates of home ownership explains a significant portion of the wealth gap, as a large portion of American families' wealth consists of home equity. See Signe-Mary McKernan, Caroline Ratcliffe, C. Eugene Steuerle, and Sisi Zhang, *Less than Equal: Racial Disparities in Wealth Accumulation* (Washington, D.C.: Urban Institute, 2013).

13. Commonwealth Fund, "African Americans Have the Highest Rates of Medical Bills and Medical Debt."

14. W. E. B. Du Bois, *The Philadelphia Negro* (New York: Lippincott, 1899), http://media.pfeiffer.edu/lridener/dss/DuBois/pntoc.html, emphasis added.

15. Thomas A. LaVeist, Darrell J. Gaskin, and Patrick Richard, *The Economic Burden of Health Inequalities in the United States* (Washington, D.C.: Joint Center for Political and Economic Studies, 2009).

16. U.S. Congress, "National Health Program, 1949: Hearings before a Subcommittee of the Committee on Labor and Public Welfare, United States Senate, Eighty-First Congress, First Session on S. 1106, S. 1456, S. 1581, and S. 1679, Bills Relative to a National Health Program of 1949. May 23, 24, 25, 31, June 1, 2, 1949," 111, https://archive.org/stream/nationalhealthpr00unit/nationalhealthpr00unit_djvu.txt. See Rosemary A. Stevens, "History and Health Policy in the United States: The Making of a Health Care Industry, 1948–2008," *Social History of Medicine* 21, no. 3 (2008): 461–83.

17. Susan Searls Giroux, "Sade's Revenge: Racial Neoliberalism and the Sovereignty of Negation," *Patterns of Prejudice*, 44, no. 1 (2010): 3.

18. Stevens, "History and Health Policy," 474.

19. Ibid., 463–64. The Affordable Care Act does in some ways address these disparities in health insurance coverage and health care usage by racial minorities. A study conducted at the University of Maryland found that since the act's implementation in 2014, the rates of uninsured African Americans and Latinos were reduced by 7 percent, compared to 3 percent for Whites. See Jie Chen, Arturo Vargas-Bustamante, Karoline Mortensen, and Alexander N. Ortega, "Racial and Ethnic Disparities in Health Care Access and Utilization under the Affordable Care Act," *Medical Care* 54, no. 2 (2016): 140–46. While this is a welcome reduction, there is obviously a long way to go in attending to inequities in racialized health. Moreover, it is questionable whether and how the ACA will endure, as well as the costs a potential rollback will impose.

20. Henry Giroux, "Reading Hurricane Katrina: Race, Class, and the Biopolitics of Disposability," *College Literature* 33, no. 3 (2006): 171–96. For Giroux, "Those poor minorities of color and class, unable to contribute to the prevailing consumerist ethic, are vanishing into the sinkhole of poverty in desolate and abandoned enclaves of decaying cities and rural spaces, or in America's ever-expanding prison empire." See also Giroux's "The Politics of Disposability," *Dissident Voice*, September 1, 2006, http://www.dissidentvoice.org/.

21. Minorities are effectively excluded from the arena of pastoral public health, by which we refer to a health care system that tends to the population and protects their welfare.

22. See Rinaldo Walcott, "Zones of Black Death: Institutions, Knowledges, and States of Being," 2014 Antipode AAG Lecture, *Antipode Foundation,* http://antipodefoundation.org/.

23. Also see Harriet A. Washington, *Medical Apartheid: The Dark History of Medical Experimentation on Black Americans from Colonial Times to the Present* (New York: Anchor, 2008), for a wide-ranging study. Also see Troy Duster, *Backdoor to Eugenics* (New York: Routledge, 2003); Alondra Nelson, *Body and Soul: The Black Panther Party and the Fight against Medical Discrimination* (Minneapolis: University of Minnesota Press, 2011); and Dorothy Roberts, *Fatal*

Invention: How Science, Politics, and Big Business Re-create Race in the Twenty-First Century (New York: New Press, 2012).

24. See Dorceta Taylor, *Toxic Communities: Environmental Racism, Industrial Pollution, and Residential Mobility* (New York: New York University Press, 2014); and Sarah E. L. Wakefield and Jamie Baxter, "Linking Health Inequality and Environmental Justice: Articulating a Precautionary Framework for Research and Action," *Environmental Justice* 3, no. 3 (2010): 95–102.

25. Michael K. Brown, Martin Carnoy, Troy Duster, and David B. Oppenheimer, *Whitewashing Race: The Myth of a Color-blind Society* (Berkeley: University of California Press, 2003).

26. *Parents Involved in Cmty. Sch. v. Seattle Sch. Dist. No. 1*, 551 U.S. 701 (U.S. 2007).

27. For some examples, see Peter C. Austin, Muhammad M. Mamdani, David N. Juurlink, and Janet E. Hux, "Testing Multiple Statistical Hypotheses Resulted in Spurious Associations: A Study of Astrological Signs and Health," *Journal of Clinical Epidemiology* 59, no. 9 (2006): 964–69. Pisces did not have increased heart failure: data-driven comparisons of binary proportions between levels of a categorical variable can result in incorrect statistical significance levels.

28. Dorothy E. Roberts, "Is Race-Based Medicine Good for Us? African American Approaches to Race, Biomedicine, and Equality," *Journal of Law, Medicine, and Ethics* 36, no. 3 (2008): 537–45.

29. Robert Westley, "The Accursed Share: Genealogy, Temporality, and the Problem of Value in Black Reparations Discourse," *Representations* 92, no. 1 (2005): 81.

30. Alyosha Goldstein, "Finance and Foreclosure in the Colonial Present," *Radical History Review* 118 (2014): 54.

31. Saidiya Hartman and Stephen Best, "Fugitive Justice," *Representations* 92, no. 1 (2005): 7.

32. Goldstein, "Finance and Foreclosure," 56.

33. Saidiya V. Hartman. *Scenes of Subjection: Terror, Slavery, and Self-Making in Nineteenth-Century America* (New York: Oxford University Press, 1997), 131.

34. Ibid., 133.

35. Goldstein, "Finance and Foreclosure," 56.

36. For example, American Indian/Alaskan Natives and Blacks are more likely to forego filling their prescriptions than other racial and ethnic groups. Given the disproportionately high rates of poverty among these two groups, the cost of drugs—even when individuals have some form of health insurance—may be seen as either prohibitive or not worth the sacrifices that would have to be made to purchase other essentials (Commonwealth Fund, "African Americans Have the Highest Rates of Medical Bills and Medical Debt"). Given the amount of resources devoted to developing race-based pharmaceuticals, individuals who are

prescribed these drugs may have to make difficult decisions regarding whether these drugs are essential to their well-being, thus risking either putting themselves at greater risk healthwise if they forego the medication or jeopardizing the well-being of their finances if they decide to fill their prescriptions regularly.

37. "Inner-city" hospitals, especially those that are publicly funded, are often the place where large portions of Black individuals and families seek their health care. Since the 1990s, studies have shown that the demographics of the community that a hospital is located within—particularly the proportion of the population that is minority—plays a significant role in its eventual closure or the eventual closing of its emergency department. See Renee Y. Hsia, Arthur L. Kellermann, and Yu-Chu Shen, "Factors Associated with Closures of Emergency Departments in the United States," *JAMA* 305, no. 19 (2011): 1978–85; Renee Y. Hsia, Tanja Srebotnjak, Hemal K. Kanzaria, Charles McCulloch, and Andrew D. Auerbach, "System-Level Health Disparities in California Emergency Departments: Minorities and Medicaid Patients Are at Higher Risk of Losing Their Emergency Departments," *Annals of Emergency Medicine* 59, no. 5 (2012): 358–65; Michelle Ko, Jack Needleman, Kathryn Pitkin Derose, Miriam J. Laugesen, and Ninez A. Ponce, "Residential Segregation and the Survival of U.S. Urban Public Hospitals," *Medical Care Research and Review* 71, no. 3 (2014): 243–60. See also Ehlers and Krupar in this volume.

38. Sharona Hoffman "'Racially-Tailored' Medicine Unraveled," *American University Law Review* 55 (2005): 386.

39. See Jonathon Kahn, "How a Drug Becomes 'Ethnic': Law, Commerce, and the Production of Racial Categories in Medicine," *Yale Journal of Health Policy, Law, and Ethics* 4, no. 1 (2004), article 1, http://digitalcommons.law.yale.edu/; and Anne Pollock, *Medicating Race: Heart Disease and Durable Preoccupations with Difference* (Durham, N.C.: Duke University Press, 2012). Also see Pollock in this volume.

40. Dorothy Roberts "'What's Wrong with Race-Based Medicine?' Genes, Drugs, and Health Disparities," *Minnesota Journal of Law, Science, and Technology* 12, no. 1 (2011): 1–21. See also, for example, Pamela Sankar and Jonathan Kahn, "BiDil: Race Medicine or Race Marketing," *Health Affairs* 24 (2005): 455–63.

41. AHRQ, U.S. Department of Health and Human Services, "Disparities in Healthcare Quality among Racial and Ethnic Minority Groups: Selected Findings from the 2010 National Healthcare Quality and Disparities Report," Fact Sheet, Publication 11-0005-3-EF, http://www.ahrq.gov/.

42. Ann Morning, *The Nature of Race: How Scientists Think and Teach about Human Difference* (Berkeley: University of California Press, 2011), 110.

43. See Kathleen J. Fitzgerald, "The Continuing Significance of Race: Racial Genomics in a Postracial Era," *Humanity and Society* 38 (2014): 49–66. Regarding race-focused genomics, see Catherine Bliss, *Race Decoded: The Genomic Fight*

for Racial Justice (Palo Alto, Calif.: Stanford University Press, 2012), as well as Bliss in this volume. On the uptake of race-focused genomics in the public domain, see John Hartigan Jr., "Is Race Still Socially Constructed? The Recent Controversy over Race and Medical Genetics," *Science as Culture* 17, no. 2 (2008): 163–93; and Nikolas Rose, "Race, Risk, and Medicine in the Age of 'Your Own Personal Genome,'" *Biosocieties* 3, no. 4 (2008): 423–39. It is important to note that in racial genomics, researchers often have a nonreductive understanding of race. They might indeed see the importance in social and environmental determinants in health. These, however, are often treated simply as triggers of underlying biology. Disease is thus seen as a problem of the body in molecular medicine: and how the body responds to external stimuli is viewed as more important than the stimuli themselves. For discussion of this point, see, for instance, Jonathan Xavier Inda, *Racial Prescriptions: Pharmaceuticals, Difference, and the Politics of Life* (Burlington, Vt.: Ashgate, 2014), 107.

44. See Nikolas Rose *The Politics of Life Itself: Biomedicine, Power, and Subjectivity in the Twenty-First Century* (Princeton, N.J.: Princeton University Press, 2007), 430; and Michael Omi, "'Slippin' into Darkness': The (Re)Biologization of Race," *Journal of Asian American Studies* 13, no. 3 (2010): 343–58, esp. 346.

45. For a representative but by no means exhaustive sample, see Sander Gilman, *Difference and Pathology: Stereotypes of Sexuality, Race, and Madness* (Ithaca, N.Y.: Cornell University Press, 1985); Ian F. Haney López, *White by Law: The Legal Construction of Race* (New York: New York University Press, 1996); Michael Omi and Howard Winant, *Racial Formation in the United States: From the 1960s to the 1980s* (New York: Routledge, 1986); Tukufu Zuberi, *Thicker than Blood: How Racial Statistics Lie* (University of Minneapolis: University of Minnesota Press, 2001); Frantz Fanon, *Black Skin, White Masks*, trans. Charles Lam Markmann (New York: Grove Press, 1967); David Theo Goldberg, "The Semantics of Race," *Ethnic and Racial Studies* 15 (1992): 543–69; Henry Louis Gates Jr., *Figures in Black: Words, Signs, and the "Racial" Self* (New York: Oxford University Press, 1987); Kimberlé Crenshaw, "Beyond Racism and Misogyny: Black Feminism and 2 Live Crew Controversy," in *Words that Wound: Critical Race Theory, Assaultive Speech, and the First Amendment,* ed. Mari J. Matsuda, Charles R. Lawrence III, Richard Delgado, and Kimberlé Crenshaw (Boulder, Colo.: Westview Press, 1993), 111–16; Patricia J. Williams, *The Alchemy of Race and Rights: Diary of a Law Professor* (London: Virago Press, 1993); and Ann Laura Stoler, *Race and the Education of Desire: Foucault's History of Sexuality and the Colonial Order of Things* (Durham, N.C.: Duke University Press, 1995). Within such a position, race is understood to be a notoriously difficult topic of discussion. As many critical race scholars have noted, this is because race itself is evasive. For Angela James, "While it is a *dynamic* phenomena rooted in political struggle, it is commonly observed as a *fixed* characteristic of human populations;

while it does not exist in terms of human biology, people routinely look to the human body for evidence about racial identity; while it is a biological *fiction,* it is nonetheless a social *fact."* James, "Making Sense of Race and Racial Classification," in *White Logic, White Methods: Racism and Methodology,* ed. Tukufu Zuberi and Eduardo Bonilla-Silva (Lanham, Md.: Rowman & Littlefield, 2008), 32.

46. Ian Haney López, "The Social Construction of Race," in *Critical Race Theory: The Cutting Edge,* ed. Richard Delgado and Jean Stephancic (Philadelphia, Pa.: Temple University Press, 2000), 165.

47. Ibid.

48. Troy Duster, "Medicine and People of Color: Unlikely Mix—Race, Biology, and Drugs," *San Francisco Chronicle,* March 17, 2003, http://www.sfgate.com/.

49. Kelly E. Happe, "The Rhetoric of Race in Breast Cancer Research," *Patterns of Prejudice* 40, no. 4–5 (2006): 467.

50. See Ehlers and Krupar in this volume.

I
RACE-BASED MEDICINE AND
MONETARY DEBT

1

The High Cost of Having Hypertension while Black in America

LESLIE R. HINKSON

Although officially over as of 2009, the Great Recession, the most damaging economic crisis since the Great Depression, has left a lasting imprint on the global economy as a whole and on the financial, political, and social landscape of American society in particular. It has been credited with a record number of foreclosures and bankruptcies, a rise in the rate of homelessness, high rates of long-term unemployment, a significant shrinking of the middle class, and an increase in the wealth and income gaps between the wealthy and everyone else.[1]

Less advertised but equally as important is the disproportionate effect the economic downturn has had on the fortunes of non-Whites in the United States. While Americans from all walks of life were negatively affected by the Great Recession, the nation's Black and Brown populace was even more so. For example, from 2007 to 2009, the net worth of Latino and Black households dropped 66 and 53 percent, respectively. The net worth of White households dropped 16 percent.[2] And while unemployment peaked at 16 and 13 percent for Blacks and Latinos, respectively, during this period, the rate of White unemployment peaked at 9.3 percent. Furthermore, although Blacks made up 12 percent of the labor force in January 2012, they made up almost 24 percent of those unemployed for a year or more.[3]

The causes of the Great Recession have been debated since 2007 and will be debated for some time to come. However, most experts agree that one factor played a significant role: debt. The housing bubble, which burst in 2007, led to a high rate of defaults on subprime mortgages. Exposure to these bad mortgages led to the collapse of some financial institutions and the near-collapse of others. The expansion of a debtor class led at first to unprecedented profits for those who created the debt in the first place. But when those debts were not able to be collected, the cumulative effect of that loss reverberated across the U.S. economy.

This expansion of lending was seen, at least at first, as laudable and a positive legacy of the Clinton administration. For too long, too many individuals and families were excluded from the American Dream of homeownership as a result of a history of discriminatory lending practices. In the rush to expand markets and to maximize profits, however, the rhetoric of inclusion was used as a justification to further extend loans to those who could not afford to repay them, a practice made possible by the Clinton administration's simultaneous sweeping deregulations of the banking and mortgage industries. Even more worrying, this rhetoric was used as cover for companies that offered unfavorable loan conditions for potential lenders—not based on their credit history but based on their race. These seemingly disconnected arms of domestic policy ushered in an expansion of predatory lending practices that disproportionately targeted minority households and ensured their inability to repay these loans. This was true not just for those who lacked the resources to own a home but also for many households that qualified for prime mortgages and were at low risk for defaulting on the terms of such lending agreements, but whose race and zip code set them up for financial failure in the predatory subprime mortgage market.

Around the same time that the United States' financial and government institutions were creating the conditions necessary for the Great Recession, another tale of profits and losses was unfolding. The fields of bioscience and medicine were becoming increasingly profit oriented. In the hunt for profits, the need to expand existing markets and find new ones became a top priority. The mapping of the human genome, biomedicine's mission to use the former's knowledge to offer individualized medicine, and the disturbing rise in the focus on race as biological truth in extending both endeavors offered a novel way to segment the market for biomedical technologies. Might different racial and ethnic groups be considered specialized markets?

As with the mortgage markets that preceded the Great Recession, products developed specifically for non-White consumers could potentially come with a racial tax. That is, the drugs marketed to minorities, because they were tailor made, might be more expensive than drugs used to target similar ailments in Whites. Yet while the use of race to determine access to capital would be seen as discriminatory once the practice was made public (and even led to the censure of many leading financial institutions), its use to determine access to certain technologies of care, including pharmaceuticals, has gone largely unquestioned, and when it is noted, it has often been lauded as a necessary approach to ensuring appropriate care and to reducing disparities in health outcomes.

As with the subprime mortgage crisis, the rhetoric of inclusion was co-opted by the biomedical industry and its budding arm of ethnopharmacogenomics from advocates for minority health. Just as lending institutions used race as a factor in determining the terms of many of the mortgages they underwrote before the bursting of the housing bubble called into question the financial and moral integrity of this practice, biomedical researchers increasingly turned their attention to developing drugs that targeted specific racial groups. Even if we take as a given that the intentions of those engaged in this project were pure and solely focused on providing the best medicine to those in need of it, their scientific and even ethical rightness invites questioning. Is race-based medicine an innovative approach toward eradicating health disparities? Is it grounded in scientific fact? What are the moral implications of this practice? Will its financial benefits accrue to all or simply to a select few? Does its rhetoric of inclusion mask the very real possibility that, like the subprime mortgage crisis, race-based decision making and treatments will create new health-related financial debt for minorities?

While much of the conversation surrounding race-tailored pharmaceuticals has focused on the drug BiDil, there exist quite a few drugs for an array of health conditions that have been allotted a racial character by medical practitioners and health insurance companies for some time. As quiet as it's kept, race-based medicine is not a new practice, at least not where pharmaceutical interventions are concerned. For decades, certain drugs, while not developed for a specific racial group, have been disproportionately prescribed to or withheld from specific races. Perhaps the most cogent example is found in recommendations for the pharmacological treatment of hypertension, or sustained elevated blood pressure. While national guidelines have suggested that race be considered in selecting appropriate drug therapies for the disease, such guidelines have also stated that race should not be used as a primary or definitive factor in their use.

How does this tie into issues of debt, especially monetary debt? I contend that not only have doctors used race as a primary factor in the drugs they select for treating hypertension, but also that drugs are often prescribed in racialized patterns that are inconsistent with treatment guidelines. These deviations from national guidelines place Black patients in particular at higher risk of greater medical costs. These costs may come directly from being prescribed more expensive medications than their White counterparts; from poorer health outcomes that are a direct result of racialized care that goes against national guidelines for treatment of hypertension; and from greater levels of health-related debt as a result of the two.

Race-based Medical Decision Making

As noted in this volume's introduction, "race-based medecine" "can be defined as the systematic targeting of racial groups for special consideration when diagnosing certain ailments or treating certain diseases." Medical decision making at the practitioner level comprises a small but integral component of that system. Researchers writing of race-based decision making in medicine tend to identify two main processes that guide it—what I have previously termed racial profiling and racial valuation.[4] I define racial profiling as "the use of race as a rationale for differential treatment of patients on the basis of predictions regarding prevalence of complications and response to specific therapies."[5] Racial profiling in medicine is thus a form of statistical discrimination. Racial valuation, on the other hand, is "defined as a process by which newer, more expensive, and/or more complex and comprehensive treatment regimens and procedures are provided disproportionately to individuals located at the top of the racial hierarchy, while those below are offered these goods and services at much lower rates."[6] Regardless of which of these processes comes into play, patients subject to race-based decision making are at risk for paying more for treatments that fit their racialized identity but that may not fit their individual health needs.

One could posit that Blacks in America have historically received less for more than many other U.S. citizens. The housing market is one case in point. A study published by the U.S. Department of Housing and Urban Development in 2011 showed that on average, White households pay less rent than African American households; that across at least ten metropolitan statistical areas (MSAs) African Americans pay a rent premium to inhabit housing of equal quality and in similar neighborhoods as their White counterparts; and that African Americans pay more to live in low-poverty neighborhoods than their White counterparts.[7] Even before the recent subprime mortgage crisis, researchers documented that many Black households received less favorable lending terms than Whites with similar credit scores and loan-to-value ratios.[8] Interestingly, Wyly and

Ponder show that inequalities in predatory subprime lending practices are intensified when we concentrate on the intersection of race and gender, particularly the experiences of Black women.[9] That is, Black women seeking home loans are disproportionately offered subprime mortgage products regardless of their income, credit score, and ability to repay. Black women are thus more likely than their White and male counterparts to be perceived or framed as credit risks and thus offered less favorable terms of repayment.

Similar trends are evident in the realm of health care. For quite some time, much of the conversation concerning health disparities and the role of institutionalized health care focused on issues of access. While Black individuals and families are still less likely to have health care coverage than their White counterparts, recent expansions of Medicaid, Child Health Insurance Plans (CHIP), and the passage of the Affordable Care Act have helped reduce the health care coverage gap over the past three decades. Health coverage in and of itself, however, does not guarantee access to care. As recent research has brought to light, the expansion of means-tested health insurance programs often coincides with a substantial decrease in the number of practices and practitioners who accept such coverage.[10] Even when Blacks have employer-based or privately paid insurance, access to care within their communities is often limited, as Blacks continue to reside in racially segregated neighborhoods and those neighborhoods continue to experience shortages in terms of health care providers within their boundaries.[11]

Issues of access aside, Blacks are also subject to different treatment when they do manage to access care. A growing body of research on race and health care focuses on the medical encounter and how racialized processes of medical decision making and rationing contribute to health disparities. For example, White physicians have been documented as spending less time with their Black patients on planning treatment, providing health education, chatting, assessing patients' health knowledge, and answering questions than with their White patients.[12] Some of this difference has been attributed to patient–doctor concordance—that is, the more similar the characteristics of patient and doctor, the more comfortable the doctor feels with the patient (and vice versa), and the greater the ease of communication.[13] Still other studies see these differences as indicative of stereotypes doctors may hold of Black patients, regardless of level of education and/or socioeconomic status, which distinguish Blacks as less able to understand detailed, technical medical advice or to be helpful partners in their own care and treatment.[14] In these cases of differential treatment, physician time and medical knowledge are rationed such that Whites receive more of both as part of their treatment. In others, specific technologies and procedures appear to be rationed such that Blacks are less likely to receive or be recommended for more advanced and expensive ones than comparable White patients.[15] Studies also document less advanced and/or less desirable technologies and procedures being recommended disproportionately for Black patients.[16]

To date, few studies have focused on racial disparities in costs for medical treatment. However, many studies have found that Blacks are less likely to receive many types of medical services and procedures. To the extent that this form of racial rationing translates into inadequate care, Blacks are thus at increased risk for complications that could otherwise have been ameliorated or prevented altogether. Inadequate care for a primary ailment may thus often lead to future complications and further ailments that incur greater costs, both monetary and physical, for Black patients.

Race-based Decision Making and Medical Error

In 2008, medical errors—which include incomplete or inaccurate diagnosis or treatment of disease, injury, syndrome, behavior, infection, or ailment—cost the United States $19.5 billion. Almost 90 percent ($17 billion) were directly associated with additional medical costs, which included ancillary services, prescription drug services, and inpatient and outpatient care.[17] While there is little in the literature documenting this, race-based decision making is a potential contributor to medical errors and their associated costs each year.

As noted above, most of the literature on race-based treatment decisions tends to focus on two primary processes: racial profiling and racial valuation. With the former, health practitioners make care and treatment decisions for individual patients based in large part on population-level risk profiles. For example, an obstetrician would be more likely to order a test for the sickle cell trait in an expectant mother who self-identifies or in some cases presents as Black than for a woman of a different race because Blacks in the United States are more likely to carry the trait than other racial groups. By the same token, a cardiovascular specialist may be less likely to prescribe beta-blockers to Black patients because the literature suggests that as a group, they may be less responsive to this medication than to other medications and more likely to exhibit adverse side effects than patients of other races. So racial profiling is in essence a form of statistical discrimination in which probabilities of the presence of certain diseases and the biological responses of individuals to treatment are predicated on race-based population-level risk profiles and help drive what treatments are offered to or denied patients. While this process may provide a quick shortcut to doctors who are increasingly under pressure to treat more patients with less time per patient visit, it sometimes results in patients being misdiagnosed, being offered the wrong treatment, or walking away without a diagnosis at all because their racial classification often overshadows their symptoms and leaves doctors stymied.

Researchers focusing on racial valuation note a different decision-making process. In this case, a different market or moral value is assigned to individuals on the basis of their racial designation. This value is based on cognitive biases and stereotypes that relate directly to racial status and the position within the social hierarchy that this status implies. So medical practitioners whose decision making is guided by this process would be more likely to provide newer, more expensive, and/or more complex and comprehensive treatment regimens and procedures to individuals located at the top of the racial hierarchy, while those below are less likely to be offered these same goods and services. It is essentially a rationing mechanism that uses race as a means of determining who gets the best and who gets the least. Treatments that are thus guided offer the potential for both undertreating patients at the bottom of the hierarchy and overtreating those at the top; both can lead to increased risk of medical error and increased medical costs.

Because race is woefully undertheorized in biomedical research and practice, using race as a guide for diagnosing and/or treating patients can often lead to medical error, which imposes both direct and indirect costs on individuals, communities, and society as a whole. Yet race is used as a diagnostic and treatment guide for a host of ailments. Treatment for hypertension is one of the most explicit examples in medical practice. An examination of treatment patterns for the disease offers a cogent illustration of how race-based treatment can lead to greater costs for Black patients. Are Black patients more likely to be prescribed the least expensive, cutting-edge treatments? Does this accord with national guidelines for the treatment of the disease? If not, how might this lead to an increased health-related debt burden for Blacks? Might assessing the ways that race-based medical decision making contributes to higher medical costs for Black patients help us better understand broader systemic influences that conspire to maintain racial wealth inequality within our society and Blacks as a debtor class for a long time to come?

Hypertension and Race-based Treatment

One of the ways that doctors try to minimize medical error is by following a model of evidence-based medical practice. This means integrating individual clinical experience and expertise with the best external evidence available to help guide practice.[18] In terms of the latter, nationally established guidelines for treatment are generally seen as the reference standard for integrating the best external evidence and distilling them into clear and concise recommendations for treatment.

For over thirty years, the National Heart, Lung, and Blood Institute (NHLBI) has coordinated guidelines designed to increase the awareness, treatment, and control of hypertension. These guidelines are widely disseminated among practitioners and researchers who are focused on cardiovascular health and disease. While these guidelines at no time recommended that race be the single most important deciding factor in selecting treatment for hypertension, their suggestion that race be taken into account may have had a significant effect in the racialized pattern of pharmacological treatment for the disease over time.

Beginning in 1984, with its Third Report of the Joint National Committee on Detection, Evaluation, and Treatment of High Blood Pressure (JNC III), the NHLBI began listing Black patients as a "special population"—the only racial group designated this status—and suggested that they responded better to diuretics than to beta-blockers.[19] In 1988, with its fourth report (JNC IV), the JNC not only repeated this recommendation but directly compared Black hypertensive patients with their White counterparts, stating that the former group did not respond as well as Whites to beta-blockers or angiotensin-converting enzyme (ACE) inhibitors.[20] The JNC V, released in January 1993, echoed these prior recommendations, pressing for research examining whether other racial and ethnic groups responded differently than Whites to treatment for hypertension.[21] In subsequent JNC reports, however, Blacks remained the single group singled out for special consideration, if not for explicitly different treatment.[22]

How a patient's race should be determined is not included in these guidelines; nor is it clear that medical practitioners have a coherent and consistent means of determining a patient's race in order to use that information to aid their diagnosis and treatment. Thus, although to date race has been discredited as a valid biological concept, we continue to use it as a crude proxy for genetic differences and for disease risk between populations.[23] How we define and measure that proxy differs across societies. For example, in the United Kingdom, recommended guidelines for hypertension treatment mirror those presently found in the United States—Blacks respond as well as Whites to monotherapy (that is, treatment with just one drug) with diuretics and calcium channel blockers (CCBs), whereas they respond less well to monotherapy with drugs that suppress the renin–angiotensin system (i.e., beta-blockers and ACE inhibitors). In the United Kingdom, however, guidelines for treatment of mixed-race individuals do not differ from those for "Whites, Asians, or Chinese" individuals.[24] There is no mention of mixed-race individuals in U.S. guidelines. The different racial taxonomies of these two societies dictate different guidelines for how race matters when treating hypertension. In the United States, how Black must an individual be before beta-blockers are dismissed as a treatment option? This use of race as a stand-in for known levels of risk and/or levels of drug metabolization, as well as the unscientific way this concept is used in the medical encounter, opens the door to medical error.

Here I use data from the Third National Health and Nutrition Examination Survey (NHANES III), conducted by the National Center for Health Statistics from 1988 to 1994 to provide a basis for distinguishing between different medical decision-making processes that produce racialized patterns in the pharmacological treatment of hypertension as opposed to providing an explanation of current trends in the prescription of hypertensive medications—hence the historical data.[25] While more recent large-scale surveys are available to researchers, the time period in which the NHANES III data were collected is interesting for a few reasons. First, it overlapped with the publication of the JNC reports that began documenting differences in response to pharmacological treatment for Blacks compared to Whites. By focusing on a period in which the acceptance of race-based recommendations for treatment were encoded in national guidelines, this study provides insight into subsequent racialized treatment patterns, as one might argue that much in medicine is path dependent,[26] and while innovation and change constantly occur in the field, these processes are influenced by self-reinforcing mechanisms that propel the existing path of knowledge creation and development.[27] Second, this was also a period in which new and relatively expensive drug treatments that we take for granted today were just being rolled out and existed for the first time alongside older, less exciting, and much less expensive drug treatments. Third, as there is generally a time lag between the publication of treatment recommendations and their acceptance and implementation by physicians, the introduction of special treatment regimens for Blacks in 1984 provided ample time for physicians in the NHANES III data collection phase (four to ten years) to modify their prescription patterns accordingly.

NHANES III is a cross-sectional, stratified multistage probability sample of the civilian noninstitutionalized U.S. population with an oversample of several population segments, including non-Hispanic Black respondents. Data were collected in household interviews, detailed clinical examinations, and laboratory tests (National Center for Health Statistics 1994).[28] The analytic sample I use here was restricted to non-Hispanic White and Black adults aged twenty-five to seventy-five years with doctor-diagnosed hypertension and valid education information (N = 3,103). All NHANES respondents were asked, "Has your doctor ever said you had high blood pressure?" An affirmative answer to this question was an indicator of diagnosed hypertension.

Univariate and bivariate statistical analyses were used to assess the distribution of key variables among White and Black men and women, as well as differences across these groups. Logistic sex-stratified models were used to estimate the effect of race on the odds of being prescribed a specific antihypertensive medication class. Because a large portion of the sample was on two or more antihypertensive medications, this necessitated estimating separate models for each medication class. Models including the full sample were also constructed using sex-by-race dummies. All descriptive and multivariate analyses were adjusted for sampling weights and the complex sampling design. The results, discussed below, indicate a racialized pattern of treatment for hypertension. They also raise questions about the subsequent costs of such treatment. Does it cost more to be treated for hypertension if you are Black in the United States? How might a discussion of differential costs provide added insight into broader discussions of race- and health-related monetary debt?

Race-based Treatment and Disparate Costs

Table 1 summarizes the distribution of key variables by race and sex. Black adults were younger, had less education, and were less likely to be insured than Whites. In the full sample, about a quarter of adults reported having been told by a doctor that they had hypertension; however, the proportion was somewhat higher among Black men and women than their White counterparts.

Table 1. Distribution of select sample characteristics, White and Black adults age 25–75: Third National Health and Nutrition Examination Survey.

	White men	White women	Black men	Black women	Difference[1]
N	2,684	3,089	1,907	2,242	
Age—mean (s.e.)	45.5 (.4)	46.3 (.5)	42.8 (.3)	43.4 (.5)	***
Education—mean (s.e.)	13.0 (.1)	12.8 (.1)	11.6 (.1)	11.8 (.1)	***
South	32.7	31.6	54.5	52.4	***
Non-metro area	54.8	56.8	42.2	41.2	**
Not married	21.0	29.6	42.5	57.8	***
Health insurance[2]	91.1	92.1	84.8	87.2	***
Reported HBP[3]	24.0	24.5	27.8	34.8	***
Measured HBP[4]	19.9	14.3	25.8	22.6	***
Any antihypertensive med.	49.9	57.4	49.2	60.5	***
Number of antihypertensive medication[5]					***
0	50.1	42.6	50.8	39.5	
1	30.0	36.2	29.3	35.5	
2	14.4	17.1	13.3	18.4	
3+	5.5	4.2	6.6	6.5	
Specific antihypertensive medication					
Diuretics	14.2	27.3	19.7	29.2	***
Calcium blockers	17.8	14.2	19.8	23.5	**
Beta blockers	17.4	18.4	10.8	11.2	**
ACE inhibitors	16.8	14.2	14.0	15.1	n.s.
Other	9.7	9.1	13.2	14.2	**
Combination therapy	19.9	21.2	19.9	24.9	n.s.
Comorbidities					
Diabetes	5.0	5.3	6.2	9.8	***
Heart failure	2.1	1.5	2.8	2.5	**
Obesity	21.3	24.3	21.6	39.0	***
Plasma levels of—mean (s.e.)					
Sodium (mmol/L)	141.3 (.1)	140.8 (.2)	141.3 (.2)	141.0 (.2)	**
Calcium (mmol/L)	2.3 (.0)	2.3 (.0)	2.3 (.0)	2.3 (.0)	n.s.
Potassium (mmol/L)	4.1 (.0)	4.0 (.0)	4.0 (.0)	3.9 (.0)	***
Vitamin D (mmol/L)	80.1 (1.7)	68.2 (1.1)	52.9 (1.6)	46.1 (1.2)	***

* $p<0.1$, ** $p<0.05$, *** $p<0.01$
Note: Shown are proportions unless specified otherwise. Adjusted for sampling design.
[1] Design-adjusted Wald tests and chi-square tests are used to assess difference among the four groups.
[2] Proportion with any health insurance (public or private).
[3] Proportion who reported that their doctor told them at least once that they had high blood pressure.
[4] Proportion with systolic pressure >140 mm/Hg or diastolic > 90mm/Hg measured during examination.
[5] Proportion on any hypertensive medication of those who self-reported hypertension.

Hypertension, as measured during the survey medical examination, had lower prevalence, likely due in part to the medication the respondents were prescribed, but Black adults had higher prevalence of high blood pressure than White adults. In terms of specific pharmacological treatments, Blacks were more likely to take diuretics, CCBs, and the "other" medication class, and they were less likely to take beta-blockers. However, Black women were more likely to take ACE inhibitors than White women, while Black men were less likely than White men to receive this medication. Some of these differences could be due to comorbidities and biochemistry profile. A higher percentage of Blacks experienced heart failure and diabetes, and a considerably larger percentage of Black women were obese than White women.

Table 2 summarizes the race differences for specific antihypertensive medications net of potential confounding or mediating variables. Each coefficient in Table 2, showing the odds ratio of taking a medication for Black adults relative to White adults, is from an independently estimated model. Each line represents a specific antihypertensive medication category; each column shows a different set of control variables, from age only in model 1 to a full set of predictors in model 6.

The race differences for most medications were substantial. On the basis of JNC recommendations, differences in the use of diuretics by race were not expected. The data showed otherwise: Black men were 73 percent more likely to be taking diuretics compared to White men of the same age. This difference was not explained by a comprehensive set of possible mediators. Through model 6, the race effect gradually became stronger: all else being equal, Black men were 128 percent more likely to be taking diuretics. The race differences among women were smaller—the odds ratio, although large in substantive terms (odds ratio = 1.35 in model 1), was significantly different from zero only in the first model.

As with diuretics, racial differences in the use of CCBs based on JNC recommendations were not expected. Among men, no significant differences were found. However, Black women were more than twice as likely as White women to take CCBs, and the odds ratio did not attenuate at all once potential explanatory covariates were adjusted for.

On the basis of the JNC recommendations, Black adults should be found less likely to be prescribed beta-blockers. The data supported this expectation: Black men and women were significantly less likely to be prescribed this class of medication than their White counterparts (odds ratio = 0.65 for men and 0.61 for women in model 1). Again, the race differences strengthened as more controls were added, suggesting that

Table 2. The effect of race on the odds of getting a given drug class for hypertension, OR (95% CI).

	Model 1	Model 2	Model 3	Model 4	Model 5	Model 6
Men						
Diuretics	1.73***	1.86***	1.86**	2.01***	2.01***	2.28***
	(1.26,2.38)	(1.25,2.76)	(1.17,2.96)	(1.21,3.31)	(1.23,3.30)	(1.29,4.03)
Calcium Channel Blockers	1.29	1.26	1.29	1.35	1.39	1.42
	(0.85,1.96)	(0.82,1.94)	(0.80,2.08)	(0.82,2.24)	(0.84,2.30)	(0.83,2.44)
Beta Blockers	0.65*	0.55**	0.59**	0.60*	0.61*	0.45**
	(0.40,1.06)	(0.33,0.93)	(0.35,1.00)	(0.35,1.02)	(0.36,1.04)	(0.22,0.91)
Ace Inhibitors	0.92	0.87	0.94	0.96	0.94	0.93
	(0.62,1.38)	(0.55,1.38)	(0.59,1.50)	(0.59,1.56)	(0.59,1.49)	(0.51,1.68)
Other	1.73***	1.82***	1.75**	1.54*	1.56*	1.36
	(1.17,2.57)	(1.19,2.77)	(1.13,2.70)	(0.96,2.45)	(0.99,2.45)	(0.78,2.34)
Women						
Diuretics	1.35*	1.15	1.21	1.23	1.21	1.15
	(0.98,1.87)	(0.79,1.68)	(0.82,1.78)	(0.84,1.80)	(0.82,1.79)	(0.72,1.81)
Calcium Channel Blockers	2.30***	2.24***	2.52***	2.59***	2.53***	2.37***
	(1.56,3.39)	(1.50,3.35)	(1.62,3.93)	(1.70,3.94)	(1.66,3.86)	(1.45,3.86)
Beta Blockers	0.61***	0.51***	0.51***	0.50***	0.51***	0.55***
	(0.43,0.88)	(0.36,0.72)	(0.35,0.74)	(0.35,0.74)	(0.35,0.75)	(0.36,0.83)
Ace Inhibitors	1.26	1.14	1.23	1.25	1.21	1.11
	(0.87,1.83)	(0.78,1.65)	(0.82,1.85)	(0.84,1.87)	(0.81,1.81)	(0.72,1.71)
Other	2.09***	1.96***	1.73**	1.68**	1.66**	1.57
	(1.45,3.01)	(1.31,2.92)	(1.11,2.69)	(1.05,2.68)	(1.03,2.68)	(0.89,2.76)

Each coefficient shows the effect of being Black on the odds of taking the specific medication, estimated in a separate sex-stratified model.
Model 1 adjusts for age.
Model 2 adjusts for age and multiple antihypertensive medications.
Model 3 adjusts for above, plus demographics: region, non-metropolitan residence, and unmarried status.
Model 4 adjusts for above, plus socioeconomic indicators: education and health insurance.
Model 5 adjusts for above, plus medical conditions: diabetes, heart failure, and obesity.
Model 6 adjusts for above, plus blood serum levels of K, Ca, Na, and vitamin D.

they were not due to differences between Black and White adults in socioeconomic status, comorbidities, or blood biochemistry profile. Blacks should also be less likely to be prescribed ACE inhibitors than Whites according to the suggestions included in the national guidelines. However, the differences observed were not statistically significant. Interestingly, while the coefficients were in the expected direction of lower odds for

Black men using an ACE inhibitor, models for women suggested the opposite pattern. Finally, JNC recommendations did not mention race as a factor in prescribing drugs in the "other" medication class. Black men and women, however, were significantly and substantially more likely to use a medication from this class, with odds ratios in the first model of 1.73 for men and 2.09 for women. This class was the only series of nested models where the control variables, particularly the blood serum levels, explained the gross difference observed in model 1.

What do these findings mean in the context of my discussion here? First, they provide evidence that during the time period 1988 to 1994, medical practitioners prescribed different drugs for the treatment of hypertension on the basis of the race of the patient. Interestingly, they also show considerable sex difference in how race affects the likelihood of being prescribed particular medication types. For example, while Black men and women were both less likely to be prescribed beta-blockers, Black men were significantly more likely to be prescribed diuretics than White men, while Black women were significantly more likely to be prescribed CCBs than White women. In other words, only one drug, beta-blockers, followed prescription patterns that suggested doctors were racially profiling Black patients. On the other hand, the large racial difference in the prescription patterns of diuretics for men—the oldest, cheapest class of hypertensive drug available—suggests that Black men were systematically being treated with a drug of lower value than White men despite national guidelines stating that this was in effect a universal drug. CCBs at the time of data collection were the newest, most cutting-edge, and most expensive class of hypertensive drug on the market, and Black women were more likely to be prescribed it than White women, thus possibly turning the racial valuation model on its head. No other statistically significant differences in prescription patterns were found, suggesting that different processes of race-based medical decision making are at play when doctors treat men and women.

The second important insight is that the gross race differences across medication classes were not explained by treatment guidelines. In other words, while doctors in the sample are using race to determine treatment, its use does not seem to follow a logic that is based on national guidelines or the best external evidence for using race in an effective way. While doctors seemed to follow recommendations concerning race and the use of beta-blockers, national guidelines provide no basis for the large, highly significant racial differences in the prescription of diuretics for men and CCBs for women. This holds true even when other confounding and mediating factors, including socioeconomic status, comorbidities, and blood serum levels of key nutrients, are taken into account. That is, even when lower rates of insurance coverage; higher rates of obesity, diabetes, and heart failure; elevated blood serum levels of sodium; and possible deficiencies in blood serum levels of calcium and vitamin D were accounted for—all trends that the biomedical and epidemiological literature tell us are more prevalent in Blacks than Whites and that might help to explain racial differences in prescription patterns—the size and significance of the race coefficient in the statistical models only increase. As noted above, one of the ways that doctors try to minimize medical error is by following a model of evidence-based medical practice. These findings indicate that in the case of hypertension at the time of the study, doctors were deviating from guidelines in a way that may have potentially increased the risk of medical error, particularly in their treatment of Black patients. Increased medical error leads to greater medical costs.

Third, the findings demonstrate that in terms of direct monetary costs, Black women were disproportionately prescribed what was at the time the newest, most expensive drug. In 1995, CCBs and ACE inhibitors were the newest and most expensive classes of antihypertensive drugs. While there are good indications for their use, during the time when the data for this chapter were collected, clinical trial evidence of their efficacy (i.e., greater reduction in risk of heart disease and stroke, greater efficacy in lowering blood pressure, fewer adverse effects) was quite limited.[29] Higher rates of CCB prescription for Black women might be suggestive of doctors more aggressively treating hypertension in Black women, as the disease is often more severe in Blacks. However, analyses including blood pressure readings (data not shown) did not yield changes in the race coefficient. This could be because those receiving medication exhibit lower blood pressure readings than they would have at time of initial diagnosis. Without data on severity of hypertension at time of prescription, it is impossible to tell whether severity is what drove these racial differences among women. Even if it were, given the nature of the data, it would remain unknown whether perceptions of differences in severity were data driven or just another taken-for-granted bit of institutionalized knowledge regarding the condition of Black patients.[30] However, given that hypertension is even more severe in Black men than in White men or in women of any race, why aren't similar trends observed among men?

In any case, Black women were more likely to receive the newest drug technology for hypertension, but at a time when evidence concerning the drugs' efficacy and safety was still tenuous. A cynical observer might conclude that Black women were effectively being used as guinea pigs. Despite the potential higher risks associated with CCBs, they also carried a higher price tag. To give some idea of the price differential, average wholesale costs (note that pharmacists typically add a 40 to 50 percent markup) for the different classes of antihypertensive medications per patient-month of therapy during this time averaged $47.63 for CCBs, $36.14 for ACE inhibitors, $23.77 for beta-blockers, and $8.25 for diuretics. Within the diuretic class, costs ranged from a low of $2.01 for thiazides and a high of $12.32 for potassium-sparing diuretics.[31] The Red Book listing of drug prices for antihypertensive agents in 1992 shows differences ranging from $0.95 per patient-month of treatment with hydrochlorothiazide (a diuretic) to $80 for proprietary (nongeneric) nifedipine (a CCB).[32]

Not only were Black women being prescribed the most expensive drug to control their hypertension at the time but they were also the least financially able to absorb this cost. In 1992, Black women earned 64 cents for every dollar earned by White men. By 2007, right before the height of the Great Recession, while this figure did not change for Black women, White women would be earning 78 cents for every dollar earned by a White man.[33] In that same year, White women had a median wealth of $45,000 compared to $100 for Black women.[34] Forty-six percent of single Black mothers and 12 percent of married Black mothers live below the poverty line compared to 32 percent of single and 5 percent of married White mothers.[35] Further, given that most people with hypertension are over the age of sixty-five, Black women receive $9,825 in annual Social Security benefits compared to $10,794 for Black men, $10,917 for White women, and $14,025 for White men.[36] Given their relative lack of wealth and lower income, it is surprising that Black women would be more likely than White women to be prescribed the most expensive class of hypertensive drugs. It is also likely that the costs associated with the drug significantly squeezed their pocketbooks.

Aside from the direct costs of the drug, CCBs also required more physician follow-up visits than other drugs prescribed during this time (with the exception of ACE inhibitors). More than twenty years hence, CCBs, while no longer new, still require more frequent physician follow-ups for monitoring—and the nongenerics are still relatively costly. Why prescribe a drug that requires higher health care costs in the form of more follow-up visits with physicians as well as the higher price of the drug itself to a group that is disproportionately lower income? Some say it is because Black women are more likely to be obese and CCBs work particularly well with obese patients. Yet after controlling for obesity, I find that Black women are even more likely to be prescribed this drug than their White counterparts. Also, nothing in the guidelines for the treatment of hypertension noted specific drug therapies for comorbid hypertension and obesity. Adding to the greater costs, these data were collected before Part D of Medicare was introduced, meaning that for most research subjects (considering the high percentage over the age of sixty-five), much of the cost of prescription drugs was out of pocket. Black women were thus more likely to be hit with two forms of higher costs for their hypertension treatment in the form of higher prescription costs and the cost of more frequent doctor visits for monitoring of the drug's use.

What about Black men? As the data indicate, they were much more likely to be prescribed the oldest, least expensive drugs requiring the least amount of follow-up for treatment. Black men are more likely than their White or female counterparts to have hypertension, and they were less likely to have their hypertension under control during the time frame in which the data were collected up through the time period 2003 to 2006.[37] It should be noted that since 1994, JNC guidelines have been updated to list diuretics as the primary recommended initial pharmacologic agent for the treatment of hypertension unless compelling indications are present that dictate the use of a different drug or the use of a diuretic plus another drug. Thus, Black men seem to have been getting the best treatment, at least initially, and yet are less likely to have their hypertension under control. In the absence of longitudinal data tracking their care, it is difficult to assess why they are more likely to be prescribed this drug and the extent to which such a plan of treatment is actually effective.

Because hypertension is the most important modifiable risk factor for cardiovascular, cerebrovascular, and renal disease, if Black men are less likely to have their diagnosed hypertension under control, they are placed at higher risk for these conditions, for associated days lost from work because of these illnesses, and for higher medical bills to treat them. Thus, while prescription patterns for Black men with hypertension indicate that they incur the lowest direct costs for treatment of the disease, in the long run, especially given their higher incidence of uncontrolled hypertension, they run the risk of accruing much higher medical bills and other indirect costs associated with their health as a result of their treatment.

Race-based Decision Making and the Racialization of Color-blind Drugs

One of the possible conclusions to be drawn from these analyses is that over time, drugs initially designed for the mass market without any indications for use in a specific racial or ethnic group can adopt a racialized identity. In the case of hypertension, by 1994, we already see the identification of diuretics (as measured by prescription patterns) as the most appropriate first-line antihypertensive treatment for Blacks, and for Black men specifically. In her 2008 article on pharmaceutical meaning making, Anne Pollock notes the racialized identity that both Roland Fryer and Henry Louis Gates Jr. seemed to ascribe to hydrochlorothiazide, a diuretic.[38] Diuretics work by reducing blood volume through facilitation of sodium excretion. If the source of one's elevated blood pressure is higher blood serum levels of sodium that cannot be reduced through restricting sodium intake alone, then a diuretic is generally the best line of therapy. However, Fryer and Gates did not associate the drug with diet but with a long discredited salt-slavery hypothesis that linked a supposed predisposition for salt retention in Blacks to those who survived the Middle Passage as a result of their ability to conserve salt and thus survive the diarrheic diseases that their salt-sparing brethren could not. If a scholar like Gates, whose work cautions us against reifying race, can even jokingly identify this drug as the best treatment for "a salt-saving Negro" like himself, it should come as no surprise that doctors who are not trained to appreciate the complexities of what race is and is not would conflate a color-blind treatment with color-coded hypothesized causal pathways for the disease. That is, hydrochlorothiazides become the go-to drug to treat "salt-saving Negros" regardless of whether salt retention is what underlies their condition. In this case, Black bodies are deviant in that they retain too much of something.

In the case of beta-blockers, however, one could say that Black bodies are seen as deviant because they have too little of something. It has been hypothesized that Blacks are less responsive to beta-blockers because they are deficient in nitric oxide, plasma renin activity, or both. However, researchers have questioned whether this differential response in fact exists or is significant, as well as whether these pathways explain differential responses in the first place. In terms of whether these differences actually exist, research has highlighted the fact that Blacks and Whites respond similarly to antihypertensive drugs even when used as monotherapy agents.[39] In a review of clinical trials conducted from 1984 to 1998, Sehgal showed that not only were Blacks in these studies more likely to have higher baseline blood pressures than their White counterparts—thus possibly skewing the results to show a weaker response to certain drugs than Whites—but also that the magnitude of the Black–White differences is much smaller than the variation within each race group.[40] In other words, the so-called Black–White difference in response to pharmacological interventions is more a matter of the direction and interpretation of the clinical trial results than real, significant differences in response by race.

Brewster and Seedat conducted a meta-analysis of studies focusing on the efficacy of antihypertensive therapies in patients of African ancestry and concluded that on the basis of existing studies, considerable overlap exists in response rates to beta-blockers between races, and that the link between hypothesized lower levels of plasma renin activity or nitric oxide are either not supported by the data or what data do exist are currently unconvincing.[41] However, they contend that self-identified ethnogeographic ancestry remained the best available predictor of response to specific antihypertensive drugs. In other words, where significant differences in response to specific drugs are found, while there is no support for the existence of hypothesized racial differences in the pathogenesis of the disease, self-identified ethnogeographic ancestry remains a significant predictor. As the authors recommend, further research on the environmental factors that might be driving these responses should be undertaken. This research also suggests that more attention be paid to how and why we use these categories in biomedical research.

Regardless of whether the research convincingly illustrates racial differences in response rates and provides a compelling and supportable reason for those differences, the example of hypertension treatment in the United States shows that drugs may adopt a racial character over time even without deliberate racial packaging. This racial character may lead to a system in which some patients are given one type of treatment and others another based on a historical social construct rather than on rigorous evidence-based treatment results. If left unchecked, such practices will continue to result in the disparate accumulation of multiple forms of debt, with Blacks more often than not being the ones in the red.

Conclusion

In my example of hypertension, Blacks are treated as a biological group distinct from all other races. Their race signals either a lack of something good—for example, nitric oxide—or an abundance of something that is bad—for example, the higher rates of obesity in Black women, or higher rates of salt sensitivity across the sexes. Most medical journal articles on hypertension and race do not discuss environment, inequality, politics, history, or discrimination. The discussion is reduced to seemingly individual-level cellular processes that are equated with one's Blackness.

As the example of hypertension shows, race-based medical decision making places Blacks at risk of facing higher medical costs than their White counterparts. This is due in part to Black women being disproportionately prescribed more expensive treatments for the same disease. Paradoxically, it is also due to Black men being prescribed the least expensive, least innovative treatments, that their ability to control their hypertension may have been reduced, thus increasing their chances of developing more serious diseases that later require more intensive and expensive treatment. In both cases, it is clear that, at least when looking at the example of hypertension, race-based medicine can significantly increase monetary costs and the risk of accumulating monetary debt for one of the least wealthy demographics in the United States—and hypertension is not the only disease or illness for which we see clear patterns of disparate treatment that potentially lead to greater monetary costs.

Cystic fibrosis is a disease that is most commonly found in Whites but affects all racial groups. In a 2003 article, a medical doctor wrote about a childhood friend who was not diagnosed with cystic fibrosis until she was eight even though she had exhibited symptoms for six years before her diagnosis. He contends the misdiagnosis stemmed from the fact that cystic fibrosis is considered a White disease—or at least not one that affects Blacks. He worries that one day a doctor will misdiagnose his daughter because the doctor may make assumptions about his daughter's race and her associated medical risk profile.[42]

Black children with asthma are significantly less likely to be prescribed treatment for their condition that follows national guidelines compared to their White counterparts. Doctors are less likely to recommend cardiac diagnostic and therapeutic procedures for Black patients.[43] Blacks also receive less pain medication than Whites for identical ailments.[44] Blacks receive less curative surgery than Whites for non–small cell lung cancer.[45] Black patients are less likely to be given physician referrals for renal transplantation.[46] The list goes on and on. While the disparities in care differ across disease type, severity of the condition, and medical specialty associated with treatment, all of these examples illustrate that race operates as a significant and independent factor in the medical decision-making process. Through relying on a race-based risk profile—and on assumptions about a patient's heredity—doctors run the risk of misdiagnosing patients, and patients are placed at risk of prolonged suffering, greater health costs and related debt, and greater mortality risk. Thus, race-based medicine generally and racialized decision making more specifically impose both direct and indirect monetary costs on Black patients as well as direct and indirect costs on their health.

There are other costs to consider as well. With the current embrace of race-based medicine, we see the reentrenchment and solidification of race as a biological reality. In the past, science was used to justify political systems that overtly advocated racial injustice. Today, such a political system seems to be part of a distant past. However, our supposedly postracial brave new world features the harnessing of our public funds through government grants to further a scientific research agenda that yields substantial rewards to those engaged in the racial project of discovering the biological reality of race. I hope that my work here inspires others to consider the price such a research agenda, its associated trends in medical treatment, and the existence of a race-based system of health care provision and delivery places on these racialized subjects and on our society as a whole.

The Great Recession provides two important lessons for those engaged in and those who support race-based medicine. Lesson one concerns the use of race as a primary criterion for service provision. In terms of the mortgage crisis, regardless of financial viability, Blacks were disproportionately targeted for unfavorable loan conditions that not only increased the probability that they would default on their mortgages but that also would place the larger economic system at increased risk. Isn't looking at an individual's wealth, income, and credit history a better indicator of ability to qualify for a prime mortgage than race? If more Black loan applicants were viewed as individuals as opposed to representatives of population-level risk profiles regarding their ability to repay a loan (not to mention their moral suitability to be afforded the trust to do so), far fewer Black households would have been the victims of foreclosure or saddled with inordinate levels of home-related debt as we see today. Such race-based lending practices hurt not just Blacks but significantly decreased the strength of the U.S. and global economies. By the same token, if race were less of a factor in not just the types of drugs that Blacks are prescribed but also in the quality and quantity of health care they are afforded, perhaps the amount of health-related debt they hold would be less significant and our nation's overall health care costs would be lower.

The second lesson concerns what appears to be the growing segmentation of the biomedical industry along racial lines. Justifying expanding markets for profit along racial lines runs the risk of exacerbating racial gaps in wealth and in levels of debt that have serious consequences for our health care system and for our economic system as a whole. If the quest for health care profits through race-based market expansion means targeting economically vulnerable groups that adds to their vulnerability, we run the risk of a zero-sum game in which the targeted group is saddled with debt and the health care system records ledger balances in the red. The mortgage crisis illustrated just that: racial and ethnic groups were targeted as ways to expand the housing market because they had been historically excluded. Now they were presented as untapped possibilities for profit. Some lenders deliberately ignored the finances of many individuals in order to make a quick profit, justifying this practice as a way to make up for the group's historical exclusion from the mortgage market. The fact that loan officers knew that some of these individuals could not possibly repay these loans illustrates the pitfalls of using race as a rationale in and of itself for creating a market niche. At the other end, many loan officers ignored the strong credit profiles of Blacks seeking mortgages and offered them home loans with unfavorable terms—terms ordinarily reserved for higher-risk borrowers. Such a practice simultaneously profiles individuals as being high risk and values them as being less deserving of favorable lending terms because of their racial affiliation. Similar trends are seen in treatment patterns for hypertension. Black men and women are simultaneously seen as at high risk for ineffectively metabolizing beta-blockers and as either being less deserving of the most innovative treatments for hypertension if male, or most deserving of the newest and least proven pharmacological treatment if female. Both avenues lead to the potential for increased rates of medical error, higher medical costs, and concomitant levels of debt for Blacks regardless of sex—and greater costs to our health care system overall.

Whether looking at housing or the health care system, Blacks are simultaneously underserved and overcharged. Until our institutions do a better job of operating with the understanding that while Blacks are a minority, they are an integral part of our economy and our society, Blacks will continue to accrue monetary debts, and our housing and health care sectors will continue to accrue ethical ones. The aftermath of the mortgage crisis revealed a moral failure on the part of our society in not holding the housing sector accountable for its ethical debts while allowing it to collect on the monetary debts it created for its victims. If we allow our health care sector to continue with its racial project of rationing care along racial lines—a practice that produces debt, inflates health care costs, and arguably increases the risk of medical error—a similar financial and ethical crisis is sure to follow.

Notes

1. David B. Grusky, Bruce Western, and Christopher Wimer, eds., *The Great Recession* (New York: Russell Sage Foundation, 2011).

2. Paul Taylor, Rakesh Kochhar, Richard Fry, Gabriel Velasco, and Seth Motel, *Wealth Gaps Rise to Record Highs between Whites, Blacks, and Hispanics* (Washington, D.C.: Pew Research Center Social and Demographic Trends, 2011), http://www.pewsocialtrends.org/files/2011/07/SDT-Wealth-Report_7-26-11_FINAL.pdf.

3. Austin Nichols and Margaret Simms, "Racial and Ethnic Differences in Receipt of Unemployment Insurance Benefits during the Great Recession," Urban Institute Unemployment and Recovery Project Brief 4, *Urban Institute*, July 23, 2012, http://www.urban.org/.

4. Leslie R. Hinkson. "The Right Profile? An Examination of Race-Based Pharmacological Treatment of Hypertension," *Sociology of Race and Ethnicity* 1, no. 2 (2015): 255–69.

5. Ibid., 258.

6. Ibid., 260.

7. Dirk W. Early, "Racial and Ethnic Disparities in Rents of Constant Quality Units in the Housing Choice Voucher Program: Evidence from HUD's Customer Satisfaction Survey," *U.S. Department of Housing and Urban Development,* 2011, https://www.huduser.gov/portal/publications/pdf/Early_RacialEthnicDisparities_AssistedHousingRCR05.pdf.

8. Debbie Gruenstein Bocian, Keith S. Ernst, and Wei Li, "Race, Ethnicity and Subprime Home Loan Pricing," *Journal of Economics and Business* 60, no. 1 (2008): 110–24.

9. Elvin Wyly and C. S. Ponder, "Gender, Age, and Race in Subprime America," *Housing Policy Debate* 21, no. 4 (2011): 529–64.

10. Peter J. Cunningham and Jack Hadley, "Effects of Changes in Incomes and Practice Circumstances on Physicians' Decisions to Treat Charity and Medicaid Patients," *Milbank Quarterly* 86, no. 1 (2008): 91–123.

11. Alan R. Nelson, Brian D. Smedley, and Adrienne Y. Stith, eds., *Unequal Treatment: Confronting Racial and Ethnic Disparities in Health Care* (Washington, D.C.: National Academies Press, 2002).

12. M. Normal Oliver, Meredith A. Goodwin, Robin S. Gotler, Patrice M. Gregory, and Kurt C. Stange, "Time Use in Clinical Encounters: Are African-American Patients Treated Differently?" *Journal of the National Medical Association* 93, no. 10 (2001): 380.

13. Lisa A. Cooper and Neil R. Powe, *Disparities in Patient Experiences, Health Care Processes, and Outcomes: The Role of Patient–Provider Racial, Ethnic, and Language Concordance* (New York: Commonwealth Fund, 2004); Jennifer Malat, "Social Distance and Patients' Rating of Healthcare Providers," *Journal*

of Health and Social Behavior (2001): 360–72; Jennifer Malat and Michelle van Ryn, "African-American Preference for Same-Race Healthcare Providers: The Role of Healthcare Discrimination," *Ethnicity and Disease* 15, no. 4 (2005): 740.

14. Rene Bowser, "Racial Profiling in Health Care: An Institutional Analysis of Medical Treatment Disparities," *Michigan Journal of Race and Law* 7 (2001): 79; Nelson, Smedley, and Stith, *Unequal Treatment*; Brian Rubineau and Yoon Kang, "Bias in White: A Longitudinal Natural Experiment Measuring Changes in Discrimination," *Management Science* 58, no. 4 (2012): 660–77.

15. See Jersey Chen, Salif S. Rathore, Martha J. Radford, Yun Wang, and Harlan M. Krumholz, "Racial Differences in the Use of Cardiac Catheterization after Acute Myocardial Infarction," *New England Journal of Medicine* 344, no. 19 (2001): 1443–49; Arnold M. Epstein and John Z. Ayanian, "Editorial: Racial Disparities in Medical Care," *New England Journal of Medicine* 344, no. 19 (2001): 1471–73; Arnold M. Epstein, John Z. Ayanian, Joseph H. Keogh, et al., "Racial Disparities in Access to Renal Transplantation: Clinically Appropriate or Due to Underuse or Overuse?," *New England Journal of Medicine* 343, no. 21 (2000): 1537–44; Nelson, Smedley, and Stith, *Unequal Treatment*; Sande Okelo, Anne L. Taylor, Jackson T. Wright Jr., Nahida Gordon, Gettha Mohan, and Edward Lesnefsky, "Race and the Decision to Refer for Coronary Revascularization: The Effect of Physician Awareness of Patient Ethnicity," *Journal of the American College of Cardiology* 38, no. 3 (2001): 698–704; Anne Pollock, "Pharmaceutical Meaning-Making Beyond Marketing: Racialized Subjects of Generic Thiazide," *Journal of Law, Medicine, and Ethics* 36, no. 3 (2008): 530–36; Dorothy Roberts, *Fatal Invention: How Science, Politics, and Big Business Recreate Race in the Twenty-First Century* (New York: New Press, 2001).

16. See Bowser, "Racial Profiling"; Scott E. Regenbogen, Atul A. Gawande, Stuart R. Lipsitz, Caprice C. Greenberg, and Ashish K. Jha, "Do Differences in Hospital and Surgeon Quality Explain Racial Disparities in Lower-Extremity Vascular Amputations?," *Annals of Surgery* 250, no. 3 (2009): 424–31; Louise Marie Roth and Megan M. Henley, "Unequal Motherhood: Racial-Ethnic and Socioeconomic Disparities in Cesarean Sections in the United States," *Social Problems* 59, no. 2 (2012): 207–27.

17. Charles Andel, Stephen L. Davidow, Mark Hollander, and David A. Moreno, "The Economics of Health Care Quality and Medical Errors," *Journal of Health Care Finance* 39, no. 1 (2012): 39–50.

18. David L. Sackett, William M. C. Rosenberg, J. A. Muir Gray, R. Brian Haynes, and W. Scott Richardson, "Evidence Based Medicine: What It Is and What It Isn't," *BMJ* 312, no. 7023 (1996): 71–72.

19. Robert M. Carey, Jeffrey Cutler, William Friedewald, et al., "The 1984 Report of the Joint National Committee on Detection, Evaluation, and Treatment of High Blood Pressure," *Archives of Internal Medicine* 144, no. 5 (1984): 1045–57.

20. Aram V. Chobanian, Michael H. Alderman, Vincent DeQuattro, et al., "The 1988 Report of the Joint National Committee on Detection, Evaluation, and Treatment of High Blood Pressure," *Archives of Internal Medicine* 148, no. 5 (1988): 1023–38.

21. Ray W. Gifford, M. H. Alderman, A. V. Chobanian, et al., "The 5th Report of the Joint National Committee on Detection, Evaluation, and Treatment of High Blood-Pressure (JNC V)," *Archives of Internal Medicine* 153, no. 2 (1993): 154–83.

22. Paul A. James, Suzanne Oparil, Barry L. Carter, et al., "2014 Evidence-Based Guideline for the Management of High Blood Pressure in Adults: Report from the Panel Members Appointed to the Eighth Joint National Committee (JNC 8)," *JAMA* 311, no. 5 (2014): 507–20; Joint National Committee on Prevention Detection, Evaluation, and Treatment of High Blood Pressure, "The Sixth Report of the Joint National Committee on Prevention, Detection, Evaluation, and Treatment of High Blood Pressure," *Archives of Internal Medicine* 157 (1997): 2413–46; Daniel W. Jones and John E. Hall, "Seventh Report of the Joint National Committee on Prevention, Detection, Evaluation, and Treatment of High Blood Pressure and Evidence from New Hypertension Trials," *Hypertension* 43, no. 1 (2004): 1–3.

23. See Lundy Braun, "Race, Ethnicity, and Health: Can Genetics Explain Disparities?," *Perspectives in Biology and Medicine* 45, no. 2 (2002): 159–74; Troy Duster, "Comparative Perspectives and Competing Explanations: Taking on the Newly Configured Reductionist Challenge to Sociology," *American Sociological Review* 71, no. 1 (2006): 1–15; Sandra Soo-Jin Lee, "Racialized Drug Design: Implications of Pharmacogenomics for Health Disparities," *American Journal of Public Health* 95, no. 12 (2005): 2133–38; Roberts, *Fatal Invention*.

24. National Collaborating Centre for Chronic Conditions (UK), *Hypertension: Management in Adults in Primary Care: Pharmacological Update* (London: Royal College of Physicians, 2006).

25. Hinkson, "Right Profile?"

26. Duster, "Comparative Perspectives"; Lee, "Racialized Drug Design."

27. Jacib S. Hacker, *The Divided Welfare State: The Battle over Public and Private Social Benefits in the United States* (Cambridge: Cambridge University Press, 2002).

28. National Center for Health Statistics, "Plan and Operation of the Third National Health and Nutrition Examination Survey, 1988–94," *Vital Health Statistics 1*, no. 32 (1994): 94–1308.

29. Teri A. Manolio, Jeffrey A. Cutler, Curt D. Furberg, Bruce M. Psaty, Paul K. Whelton, and William B. Applegate, "Trends in Pharmacologic Management of Hypertension in the United States," *Archives of Internal Medicine* 155, no. 8 (1995): 829–37.

30. Bowser, "Racial Profiling"; Lee, "Racialized Drug Design."
31. Manolio et al., "Trends in Pharmacologic Management."
32. *1992 Drug Topics Red Book* (Oradell, N.J.: Medical Economics, 1992).
33. "Closing the Wage Gap Is Crucial for Women of Color and Their Families," Fact Sheet, *National Women's Law Center*, November 2013, https://www.nwlc.org/sites/default/files/pdfs/2013.11.13_closing_the_wage_gap_is_crucial_for_woc_and_their_families.pdf.
34. Mariko Lin Chang and Meizhu Lui, *Lifting as We Climb: Women of Color, Wealth, and America's Future* (Oakland, Calif.: Insight Center for Community Economic Development, 2010).
35. Wendy Wang, Kim Parker, and Paul Taylor, "Breadwinner Moms: Pew Research, Social and Demographic Trends," *Pew Research Center*, May 29, 2013, http://www.pewsocialtrends.org/.
36. Jocelyn Fischer and Jeff Hayes, "The Importance of Social Security in the Incomes of Older Americans Differences by Gender, Age, Race/Ethnicity, and Marital Status," *Institute for Women's Policy Research*, August 2013, http://www.iwpr.org/.
37. Centers for Disease Control and Prevention, *A Closer Look at African American Men and High Blood Pressure Control: A Review of Psychosocial Factors and Systems-Level Interventions* (Atlanta, Ga.: U.S. Department of Health and Human Services, 2010), http://www.cdc.gov/bloodpressure/docs/african_american_sourcebook.pdf.
38. Pollock, "Pharmaceutical Meaning-Making."
39. Steven Epstein, *Inclusion: The Politics of Difference in Medical Research* (Chicago: University of Chicago Press, 2008).
40. Ashwini R. Sehgal, "Overlap between Whites and Blacks in Response to Antihypertensive Drugs," *Hypertension* 43, no. 3 (2004): 566–72.
41. Lizzy M. Brewster and Yackoob K. Seedat, "Why Do Hypertensive Patients of African Ancestry Respond Better to Calcium Blockers and Diuretics than to ACE Inhibitors and β-Adrenergic Blockers? A Systematic Review," *BMC Medicine* 11, no. 1 (2013): 141.
42. Richard S. Garcia, "The Misuse of Race in Medical Diagnosis," *Journal of Children's Health* 1, no. 2 (2003): 293–95.
43. See Paula A. Johnson, Thomas H. Lee, E. Francis Cook, Gregory W. Rouan, and Lee Goldman, "Effect of Race on the Presentation and Management of Patients with Acute Chest Pain," *Annals of Internal Medicine* 118, no. 8 (1993): 593–601; and Kevin A. Schulman, Jesse A. Berlin, William Harless, et al., "The Effect of Race and Sex on Physicians' Recommendations for Cardiac Catheterization," *New England Journal of Medicine* 340, no. 8 (1999): 618–26.
44. Roberto Bernabei, Giovanni Gambassi, Kate Lapane, et al., for the SAGE Study Group, "Management of Pain in Elderly Patients with Cancer," *JAMA* 279, no. 23 (1998): 1877–82; Knox H. Todd, Christi Deaton, Anne P. D'Adamo, and

Leon Goe, "Ethnicity and Analgesic Practice," *Annals of Emergency Medicine* 35, no. 1 (2000): 11–16; Knox H. Todd, Nigel Samaroo, and Jerome R. Hoffman, "Ethnicity as a Risk Factor for Inadequate Emergency Department Analgesia," *JAMA* 269, no. 12 (1993): 1537–39.

45. Peter B. Bach, Laura D. Cramer, Joan L. Warren, and Colin B. Begg, "Racial Differences in the Treatment of Early-Stage Lung Cancer," *New England Journal of Medicine* 341, no. 16 (1999): 1198–205.

46. John Z. Ayanian, Paul D. Cleary, Joel S. Weissman, and Arnold M. Epstein, "The Effect of Patients' Preferences on Racial Differences in Access to Renal Transplantation," *New England Journal of Medicine* 341, no. 22 (1999): 1661–69.

2

"When Treating Patients like Criminals Makes Sense"
Medical Hot Spotting, Race, and Debt

NADINE EHLERS AND SHILOH KRUPAR

> Imagine if you could identify a small number of patients who end up eating up most health care dollars.
> —DYLAN RATIGAN, "HOT-SPOTTING: IT'S HOW, NOT HOW MUCH" (2011)

> Over time, providers who work with high utilizers are able to categorize patients into distinct groups [one of which is described as] "socially disintegrated," [those] who tend not to engage in self-care, have few family resources and display dependent personalities.
> —HAYDN BUSH, "HEALTH CARE'S COSTLIEST 1%" (2012)

Medical hot spotting has been heralded by many as one of the most innovative recent approaches to improving health and the caregiving reach of medical professionals.[1] This practice, which began in Camden, New Jersey, in 2007, uses medical data collection, Geographic Information Systems (GIS) technologies, and spatial profiling to identify populations that are medically vulnerable in order to provide preemptive and more effective care at home. Medical hot spotting attends to the sickest of the sick: individuals who often lack health insurance and any connection to primary care providers, and individuals who have multiple and compounding chronic conditions that take them back again and again to hospital emergency departments.

Here we explore the racial contours of medical hot spotting, a focus that is particularly important given the intersections among poverty, racial minority status, and general lack of access to adequate health care. In the United States, race-based wealth inequality and the subsequent lack of access to health insurance and health care has long meant that Black individuals, among other minorities, carry an excess disease burden. In Camden, hot spotting emerged as a response to this disease burden—a means by which to address health inequalities that are regionally racialized and embodied by Camden residents. The practice of medical hot spotting is not explicitly racialized except in cases where practitioners claim to address social and environmental factors that result from the historical disenfranchisement and biomedical neglect of people of color. In this progressive sense, then, it potentially exhibits a compensatory social function to pay back an as-yet unpaid debt for historical and enduring injury and structural racism—forms of indifference, exclusion, dispossession, and violence that have produced health inequalities and Black suffering.

Importantly, however, a twin incentive of medical hot spotting is the aim of minimizing health care expenditure, specifically to lower what is known as uncompensated care debt. Those who are targeted by medical hot spotting are that 1 percent of the population who account for an excess of health care costs; precisely because these individuals have inadequate primary and preventive care and minimal or no medical insurance, their medical bills contribute to the accumulated uncompensated care debt incurred by hospitals. In much of the public discourse surrounding medical hot spotting, the imperative of cost containment and minimizing this form of health care expenditure seems to eclipse the need to attend to health inequities. This is evident in the very language used to talk about those who are targeted: they are the "high utilizers" and "the superuser 1 percent"; they are identified as "outliers" and identified as "socially disintegrated."[2] By consistently being represented in these terms, the most vulnerable are positioned as "bad" or "failed" citizens because they are presented as a drain on the U.S. health system and on society at large.

Given these factors, we take a more cautious approach to medical hot spotting. We suggest that despite being supposedly race neutral, medical hot spotting is a thoroughly racialized project. Indeed, we see it as a form of race-based medicine in the sense that it rations and rationalizes medical care and attention according to race. Rather than initiating racial redress, hot spotting actually inaugurates other, more pernicious linkages between race, health, and debt. The practice potentially supports intensified racial dominance under the auspices of improved health administration and biosecurity, and it does so largely through ontologizing racial spaces. Such speculative analysis is timely given the mounting popularity of medical hot spotting under the banner "when treating patients like criminals make sense."[3]

Before proceeding to a detailed account of the practice, however, we outline what we see as the fundamental predicates of the biomedical targeting of race. We situate medical hot spotting as a form of biomedical targeting of race that augments anti-Blackness and racial capitalism, with particularly deleterious consequences for African Americans, a population that has borne a long history of medical abuse and biopolitical neglect in the United States.

Race-Specific Biomedical Targeting

As W. E. B. Du Bois made clear as far back as the late nineteenth century, the biopolitical administration of health in the United States has been "cut"—divided and segmented—by racism.[4] Such administration must thus be seen as a race-specific biopolitics of health. Indeed, the first function of racism, Michel Foucault tells us, is "to fragment, to create caesuras within the biological continuum."[5] The "cut" of racism has meant that different segments of the population have been administered and thus governed in distinct ways and, importantly, that White lives have been affirmed and made to live in ways that Black lives have not. As Michael Dillon and Andrew W. Neal have argued, race functions as a marker that biopolitically adjudicates: race "does not only specify life's eligibilities for this or that good—it ultimately specifies whether or not a life is to be considered eligible for life as such."[6] Viewed through this lens, the differential governing or management of Black subjects both operates as a form of violence against the Black body/subject and situates African Americans as separate from the wider population and the polis. Biomedical targeting might seem to ameliorate this cut by targeting supposedly specific health factors through race-specific drugs or, in the case of medical hot spotting, by directing health care toward particular spaces to alleviate health disparities.[7] These targeting operations are deployed ostensibly to affirm life. They are said to redress past forms of biomedical neglect and enable the tailoring of biomedical intervention into vulnerable communities, and they are advocated as the means through which to foster the health of those populations—through attention, through targeting. At the same time, however, such interventions may signal inequitable and endangering forms of biomedical administration. We advance this more circumspect view through three foundational claims.

First, regardless of the motivations for biomedical targeting—that is, the will to attend to Black health—the operation of race-specific biomedical targeting of Black subjects is structured through an epistemology of anti-Blackness. More than racist actions against Blacks, or the architecture of racial discrimination, or a paradigm that binds Blackness and death together, anti-Blackness is a form of knowledge that positions the Black subject outside of the category "Human."[8] Such expulsion of Black lives from the normative position of human is undeniable, "given the histories of slavery, colonialism, segregation, lynching," and the ongoing imperiling of Black lives.[9] That biomedical targeting is structured through anti-Blackness is evident in the way it reinstitutes racial difference and separation and, as we will show, stages an additional form of violence by actually expelling Blacks from the possibility of optimal health. Black lives have been consistently threatened in and through the biomedical encounter,[10] and anti-Blackness continues to thwart Black life and futurity through biomedical targeting operations that subject African Americans to what Du Bois called a "social atmosphere . . . which differs from that surrounding whites."[11] Race-based targeting efforts that are aimed at redressing health inequities can actually recursively secure anti-Blackness by refusing to acknowledge its structuring logic, thus equating Blackness with inevitable vulnerability, risk, threat, and premature death.

Second, biomedical targeting operations extract the conditions of Black health and illness from the broader contexts of structural racism. By this, we mean that biomedical targeting generally fails to recognize the social conditions in which poor health emerges and, in the case of Black subjects, how poor health, institutional racism, and the epistemology of anti-Blackness are ontologically enmeshed. Indeed, the targeting of Black populations—specifically in the case of medical hot spotting—does not simply direct resources to Black subjects. Instead, in such operations, race is objectified as that to be targeted, meaning that race itself is thus not undone; that is, race as a stratifying mechanism that orders the social— a system characterized by anti-Blackness—is not called into question. Instead, biomedical targeting advances the epistemological violence of anti-Blackness by concentrating the "problem" of Black life in the United States at the scales of the racialized body and space (such as hot spots), which become objects of ever more heightened administration, financial exploitation or regulation, and securitization.

Third, contemporary biomedical targeting technologies are an endangering form of health administration in that they are conditioned by the logics of neoliberalism. According to Wendy Brown, neoliberalism is a governing rationality through which everything is "economized" and in a very specific way: human beings become market actors and nothing but, every field of activity is seen as a market, and every entity (whether public or private, whether person, business, or state) is governed as a firm.... Neoliberalism construes even non-wealth generating spheres ... in market terms, [it] submits them to market metrics, and governs them with market techniques and practices. Above all, it casts people as human capital who must constantly tend to their own present and future value.[12]

Importantly, neoliberal logics transform "social, cultural, and individual life.... Public institutions and services have not merely been outsourced but thoroughly recast as private goods for individual investment or consumption."[13] The neoliberal biopolitics of health increasingly emphasizes customizing health, the body, and life itself through biomedical practices.[14] Customizing health can exacerbate racial inequalities; it is inextricable from the financialization of health, it involves individualizing illness (which stresses personal responsibility and behavior), and it is predicated on implementing cost–benefit logics and the so-called color-blind agency of the free market, all of which reentrench racial domination.[15] Moreover, the decline of the welfare or pastoral state—and public health focus—has meant that the administration of life is increasingly imagined in terms of biosecurity, with heightened emphasis on preempting disease and containing high costs and so called high utilizers of the health care system. Under neoliberal conditions, populations previously projected outside of pastoral power (and excluded from the vital politics of the nation) are now being predicted, defined, and delineated in advance as risk failures and as necropolitical market opportunities.[16] Biomedical targeting technologies reveal a predatory power to demarcate race for purposes spanning from financial accumulation (seen, for instance, in the development and marketing of race-specific pharmaceuticals such as BiDil) to threat containment and the production of financial benefit (as is the case with hot spotting and the practice's goal of debt minimization). These forms of deriving or generating economic value from racial identity—what has been referred to as racial capitalism—is achieved even as such targeting is advocated as the means for addressing the embodied and spatial effects of racial inequality.[17] Moreover, the neoliberal refusal to acknowledge the social production of risk (health is an individual, not social, enterprise) and disavowal of the historical and spatial processes of racial formation that structure the present ultimately legitimates anti-Blackness and secures African American expulsion from health as the paradoxically race-neutral future of the nation.

The example of biomedical targeting that we focus on here—medical hot spotting—has not only germinated within U.S. neoliberal policy and the postreform health care landscape but has also innovatively extended neoliberal logics through race–space relations that it contradictorily renders invisible. Henry Giroux captures the rationale for our critique of the emergent practice: "Racial justice in the age of market-based freedoms and financially driven values loses its ethical imperative to a neoliberalism that embraces commercial rather than civic values, private rather than public interests, and financial incentives rather than ethical concerns."[18]

Contours of Medical Hot Spotting

The practice of medical hot spotting, as we noted earlier, began in Camden, New Jersey, an economically depressed community across the Delaware River from Philadelphia. After the collapse of its industrial base and decades of White flight, Camden is considered to be one of the most blighted areas of the northeastern United States, owing to heavy pollution from toxic industries, unsafe and abandoned structures, violent drug trade and crime, and a population of approximately 77,000 that is, per capita, one of the poorest in the nation.[19] These figures become particularly telling in light of the racial demographics of the city: according to the 2010 census, half of the city's residents were Black or African American, and more than a third of the residents were Latino.[20] Widespread industrial contamination, poverty, and escalated violent crime all contributed to a dire public health problem in Camden. With 29.5 percent of the population unable to afford prescription drugs, the city's residents clearly experience disproportionate levels of ill health.[21]

The innovations of medical hot spotting were conceived in this racialized context and have been variously defined as "the ability to identify in a timely manner heavy users of the systems and their patterns of utilization so that targeted intervention programs can be instituted"[22] and as "a problem-solving technique that *targets the most expensive problems* or in-need people by allocating resources to specific problem areas as revealed by the data."[23] The practice is attributed to Dr. Jeffrey Brenner, who founded the Camden Healthcare Providers Breakfast Group in 2002 and later the Camden Coalition of Healthcare Providers, where he serves today as full-time executive director.[24] His personal and professional interest in addressing violence in Camden led him to apply policing strate-

"WHEN TREATING PATIENTS LIKE CRIMINALS MAKES SENSE" 37

gies to health care, namely CompStat, a computer program that tracks and maps crime statistics and by so doing allows police to target areas where crimes are committed and to direct resources toward controlling these hot spots.[25] Just as such law enforcement compiles data and uses GIS technologies to identify and give special attention to areas with high crime rates, Brenner figured that a medical application—medical hot spotting—could similarly identify populations who are medically vulnerable or indigent and who are high utilizers of the health care system.[26]

Brenner reportedly obtained massive amounts of data from hospitals in the area; analyzed and mapped medical information, such as hospital readmissions and emergency department visits; and discovered that "we're wasting a lot of money in healthcare to deliver disorganized and fragmented and expensive services."[27] According to Brenner's statistics, around $100 million in health care resources had been spent on a city of under 79,000 people.[28] He found that 1 percent of the patients in Camden were driving 30 percent of the cost and that the two most expensive high-utilizing areas were a large nursing home and a low-income housing tower.[29] In different interviews, Brenner has elaborated the following statistics: "Between 2002 and 2008, nine-hundred people from those two buildings alone accounted for more than 4,000 hospital visits and $200 million in healthcare bills. A single patient had 324 hospital admissions in five years. The most expensive patient racked up $3.5 million in healthcare costs."[30] The single public housing development was alone responsible for $12 million in health care costs from 2002 to 2008.[31]

Moreover, Brenner found that people with the highest medical costs and the greatest number of emergency room visits were usually receiving the worst care. High utilizers of health care in Camden visited overburdened local clinics, were uninsured or otherwise remiss about seeing a primary care doctor for preventive care, were on welfare and otherwise poor, and were making detrimental lifestyle choices with little capacity for change, such as cycles of prescription medicine and other treatments that dealt with superficial symptoms rather than root causes of health problems.[32] A critical aspect to medical hot spotting, then, is to use this sophisticated medical data mapping to direct more efficient and effective care toward these medical hot spots of high utilizers.[33] Medical hot spotting coordinates and tailors care management through numerous techniques that restructure the organization, delivery, accountability, and doctor–patient relations of health care. These strategies include interdisciplinary teamwork, house calls and personalized follow-ups, practical preventive care rather than emergency department visits, medical escorts and transition nurses, community assistance programs, and behavioral modification techniques all focused on the individual patient over a period of up to six months.[34] Reflecting on the promise of U.S. health care reforms and medical hot spotting, Brenner has remarked, "The Patient Protection and Affordable Care Act is providing money for many demonstration programs and pilots that are intending to get similar work off the ground. Money has moved out the door for community health teams."[35] In the same interview, he has also noted, "I'm hoping that our country focuses like a laser beam on the sickest, costliest patients and doesn't misdirect all the money that is coming out of CMS [Centers for Medicare and Medicaid Services] right now and miss the opportunities."[36]

From its Camden origins, medical hot spotting has gained traction across the health care system. Similar practices are now at work in places such as Trenton, Newark, West Philadelphia, York, Scranton, Allentown, the Bronx and Queens, Atlantic City, Boston, Anchorage, Chicago, Seattle, and Las Vegas.[37] Clearly, such health care reforms and experimentations are needed social projects, and in many ways, medical hot spotting appears to be a laudatory venture, especially in terms of advocating for patient-centered care and addressing the specific health needs of the disadvantaged. At the same time, however, there are less positive and more pernicious dimensions to medical hot spotting that are both consistently reiterated in relation to the practice and not critically evaluated. Social projects such as this, we argue, are also always inherently racial projects. Indeed, the well-documented institutional racism of biomedicine, as well as the persistent forms of structural racism that underpin U.S. society and produce differential vulnerabilities to illness and disease, are part of what universal access to health care endeavors to address and even rectify.[38] Yet race remains topically out of bounds in discussions about medical hot spotting. Our contribution, then, is to consider how medical hot spotting both functions as a biomedical targeting operation and augments anti-Blackness, exposing Black subjects to heightened forms of economized social and self-management, even as practitioners and policy makers claim the practice to be race neutral.

We identify three dystopian aspects of medical hot spotting that reveal how uncompensated care debt management advances structural racism by recursively anticipating risk and debt through ontologizing racialized spaces. What we see at work, as Jenna Loyd has discussed in another context, is that "problems" are pinned "to a discrete area or group in order to define narrow programmatic, technical, or medical interventions." As she further notes, "This scaling of the problem reifies symptoms while failing to identify processes of uneven geographical development that create *interlinked* spaces of concentrated wealth and health in some places, and poverty and illness in others."[39]

From Debt to Indebtedness: Medical Hot Spotting and Enduring Conditions of Lethality

The first dystopian aspect of medical hot spotting is evident in that, although the practice aims to address the health of the medically vulnerable, it simultaneously mobilizes a national imagination of scarce health care dollars and advances a world defined by a grid of relationships of cost that fuels racial enmities.[40] The abstraction of this cost grid disregards the richness of space (the social–spatial relationships that contribute to high-cost usage of health care), and it circumscribes subjectivity within the market. Managing medical care for cost containment disregards the structural reasons for ill health by giving epistemological primacy to cost relations.[41]

Importantly, in this grid of relationships of costs, the medically vulnerable are blamed as the source of spiraling health expenditure. As such, they are interpellated as debt-producing subjects. There are countless examples of this circulating in the media: "There's a small segment that is burning through 20 percent of our society's wealth at a massive rate," or "because U.S. hospitals give billions of uncompensated care to the uninsured and under-insured each year, they pass costs along to insured users."[42] The primary debt these individuals are seen as generating—what is known as uncompensated care debt—is "an overall measure of hospital care provided for which no payment was received from the patient or insurer. It is the sum of a hospital's 'bad debt' and the charity care it provides."[43] According to the American College of Emergency Physicians, 55 percent of emergency care goes uncompensated, and according to American Hospital Association figures, national uncompensated care debt expenditure rose from $12.1 billion in 1990 to $42.8 billion in 2014.[44]

In the context of austerity policies and widespread panic about the overtaxed U.S. health care system, minimizing debt through cost efficiency amplifies a racist antagonism between those who are worthy of scarce resources—an imagined community of deserving Americans (White, suburban, healthy families)—set against the despicable, leeching high utilizers, a category that serves as proxy for racialized others. The call to locate the superuser 1 percent highlights several key factors. First, it places emphasis on patients' (seemingly unacceptable) use of services rather than focusing on their needs, as implied by the older term used for medically vulnerable individuals, "patients with complex needs." Second, it denies wider social inequities and entrenched exclusionary practices that have led to the increased use of emergency health services by disadvantaged individuals. Last, the call marshals racism by using the powerful rhetoric of statistics and unfair burden. Indeed, we may see "high utilizer" join "welfare queen" and "gangbanger" in the pantheon of demonized subjects for "endangering our national health care budget and the health of worthy citizens who are not bringing health problems on themselves."[45]

Medical hot spotting, then, easily supports the idea that hot spots (and the people within them) are a serious threat to the nation, and by locating them, it facilitates the transfer of blame and the placement of responsibility on those who are already disadvantaged and disenfranchised. This is particularly deleterious to African Americans, who have received significantly less adequate care than White Americans in the United States as a result of a host of financial, organizational, and social barriers.[46] The historically accumulated suffering of the Black body has meant African Americans are at increased risk for acute and chronic diseases, epidemics such as HIV/AIDS, and mental illness.[47] Yet the risks of Black life in America are eclipsed by racialized subjectivities that stratify the population and justify the harmful impacts of neoliberalization experienced disproportionately within racialized communities.[48] Moreover, rather than racism and conditions of lethality being viewed as killing people, individuals are viewed as killing themselves through their own actions.[49] They are viewed as risky subjects whose individual behaviors are the cause of both risk and accumulated debt. Overall, the operation of targeting the 1 percent of the U.S. health care system enacts a deeply structural logic of anti-Blackness in America, equating race, and specifically Blackness, with the antithesis of the ideal neoliberal citizen: Blackness is figured as inherently vulnerable, wasteful, unable to be self-sufficient or healthy, a burden to the nation.

If medical hot spotting recasts the question of who or what is to blame for the persistence of ill health and health care debt, then the second dystopian aspect of the practice is that it can also be said to position the medically vulnerable or indigent as indebted to the state, hospitals, and society at large, who have spent resources on them. Such a framing is possible because uncompensated debt "is shared among governments and private sponsors, although ultimately individuals bear the costs of these uncompensated services as taxpayers, providers, employees, and health care consumers."[50] Having generated this form of public expenditure, those who are disadvantaged are now positioned as being obligated to rectify this debt through the responsibilization of risk and through subsequent self-governance in order to minimize future debt accumulation. This move is evident in that medical hot spotting promotes self-care. It does so in the absence of social welfare and thus contributes to a feedback loop of racial domination.

Self-care entails a shift in biological citizenship from one who possesses rights to services to a manager of individual health risks in a context of enhanced social control and consumer access. In this context, lack of health is attributed to personal failure rather than to the structural positioning of African Americans outside of the populace. The aggregation of these failures is mapped in space for the purposes of surveillance, anticipation of risk, and containment. While autonomy and empowerment to make oneself be healthy are laudable goals, the neoliberal imperative to self-care undercuts the promise of social reform by enlisting the nation's costliest health care consumers to participate in preventive care—a process that relegates racially coded economic, social–environmental disadvantage to the private and personal spheres.[51] Neoliberal self-care asserts that individuals are solely in charge of their health and should adjust their behavior to achieve optimal health; individuals who fail to do so are bad, deviant, or even pathological subjects despite any structural issues that might preclude good health. The neoliberal logic of self-care enlists African Americans to participate as consumers of preventive care, yet it relegates any inability to do so to a private issue or racially grouped failure within a supposedly color-blind meritocracy enabled by the free market.

Medical hot spotting potentially draws attention to this neoliberal re-entrenching of anti-Blackness, specifically the way assertions of race-transcendent agency obscure structural racism. The practice seeks to intervene in the daily care of three categories of patients—the mentally ill, the medically fragile elderly, and patients who are described as socially disintegrated, or "those who tend not to engage in self-care, have few family resources and display dependent personalities."[52] The category of "socially disintegrated" seemingly offers an opportunity to examine the race-specific biopolitics of health—how poor health, institutional racism, and the epistemology of anti-Blackness are ontologically enmeshed. Anecdotal evidence and a short documentary about medical hot spotting demonstrate that medical hot spotting does attempt to expand health care into social and environmental arenas, and to cultivate social infrastructure and stability through caregiving.[53] Such efforts are undermined by the behaviorist emphasis, which medicalizes urban marginality and functionally blurs welfare and penal policies.[54] The sorting out of the so-called socially disintegrated—those who fail at/to self-care—from productive citizens allows for race to be understood as a marker of risky or dysfunctional social behaviors rather than as an indicator of racialized knowledges and experiences that make one more vulnerable.[55] One particular remark from Brenner is telling in terms of highlighting how the onus of responsibility is put onto the individual—not to mention the paternalism of the practice and how it fails to substantially address structural causes of ill health:

> The end of the intervention is determined based on hospital utilization, individual factors (health education/literacy, disease self-management, skills development, level of engagement, self-efficacy) *and some systemic factors* (access to, and the quality of, care, social support, etc.). *The person receives a graduation certificate. The person is expected to meet their healthcare needs in the future* through their primary care physician.[56]

As an intervention, medical hot spotting signals a shift in health governance and moves toward potentially more aggressive (in)voluntary programs that target individual behavior and mandate personal responsibility, just as the state is withdrawing institutional supports that are necessary to shoulder illness, unemployment, indigence, and so forth.[57] The practice could progress in the direction of racially sorting and segmenting health care to support moralizing behavioral workfare in the context of austerity and corporatized health care.[58]

The third dystopian aspect of medical hot spotting is that it risks spatially ontologizing historical geographies of racial domination (urban renewal, redlining in housing and mortgage industries, environmental racism) as simply geodemographic facts on a map, in part to manage possible future medical debt. From crime mapping and policing, medical hot spotting borrowed technologies (namely CompStat) that collect and use spatial data to model, monitor, and control criminal behaviors. First instituted by then–New York City police commissioner William Bratton in the mid-1990s, crime hot spotting generates digital cartographic representations of high-crime areas by linking statistical information such as crime type and occurrence with zip code and neighborhood.[59] Police are then able to target anticipated high-crime spaces by spatially customizing surveillance and control.[60] Similarly, medical hot spotting integrates GIS data and demographic techniques that target problem spaces and populations through spatial profiling.[61] Such geosurveillance is the logical outcome of the militarized interpretation of residents as risk factors that need to be logged, mapped, and understood in a calculative statistical manner. Medical hot spotting secures target fields of information, spatial data, and geographical identification of high-risk people and spaces for the purposes of biosecurity—that is, managing health and mitigating uncompensated care debt for the optimization of the population.[62] The auditing process—the geographical processing of medical metadata—generates a racially stratified datascape of expectations that basically reproduces what we already know. The spatial ontology at work in this targeting operation stipulates that where you are reveals who you are, as collected, assessed, and defined by marketers, governments, the police, or clinics.[63] Racialized spaces and bodies become ontologized as knowable, measurable geotags and data of a population, even when medical hot spotting does not explicitly involve racial profiling. In other words, medical hot spotting ontologizes structural racism in/as space.[64]

Medical hot spotting's application of GIS demonstrates a political rationality that calls forth surveillant uses of technology in the observation of spaces and populations, transforming governing into a field of perception.[65] The geosurveillant technologies that inform medical hot spotting arguably mobilize the ghetto as a preemptive way of seeing, of "knowing as containing."[66] Thus, establishing medical hot spots serves as a teleological spatial containment technique for the management of poverty, marginality, and health care expenditure. We could even say that identified hot spots become debt containment zones and/or spaces of supposed preknown failure: they are known as spaces that generate debt, the inhabitants are charted as debt-producing subjects, and their actions are viewed as inevitably leading to future debt generation. Such preknown risk is then managed through the hot spotting practices that we have outlined. If this is the case, what targeting the superuser 1 percent rationalizes is racially segmented care—by drawing out and further entrenching social borders and spatial segregations. In other words, minority communities might experience medical hot spotting as an intensified form of medical redlining—that is, spatially customized care as a means to ration medical resources and health care. Given the twin neoliberal imperatives of cost containment and self-care, it is not a stretch to see medical hot spotting even develop into a remote-sensored care delivery system that somatically surveils the high utilizers of health care through cost-saving home monitoring, informatizes corporeal systems to mine data, and positions bodies as nodes within a network of physiological, behavioral, and locational data connected to command centers.[67] The geosurveillant technologies of medical hot spotting reveal that health promotion and disease prevention involve increasingly militarized preemption, concentrated on preknown spaces of failure as analytic objects that can be surveilled at a distance.[68] Whether through self-responsibilization of risk or ontologizing structural racism in space, medical hot spotting reveals the future of a race-specific biopolitics of health that rationalizes and defends anti-Black biosecurity as race-neutral containment.[69]

Alternative Ethical Formations: Resituating Indebtedness

Medical hot spotting is predicated on the seemingly laudable pursuit of attending to vulnerable populations and alleviating (always already racialized) disparities of health. The operations involved in medical hot spotting potentially address specific conditions that affect Black life; they ostensibly imagine and practice a different racial future in the United States. At the same time, however, the practice is largely focused on the minimization of accumulated uncompensated care debt and future health expenditure. This goal of medical hot spotting seems to take the lead in the public arena, above and beyond the will to alleviate medical vulnerability. What such a focus elides is the reality that minorities—and particularly Blacks—have been excluded from normalized society through reduced access to employment, housing options, and health promotion and care, and that it is this exclusion that has created the problem of unwanted health care expenditure. Rather than a systematic acknowledgment of this past and enduring exclusion, however, African Americans are positioned as debt-producing subjects that are a drain on society and require intervention; the epistemology of anti-Blackness holds African Americans as having wronged society at large through supposedly being responsible for uncompensated care debt. Consequently, they are subjected to a separate form of health administration through medical hot spotting. To alleviate their debt to society, they are obligated to self-care even though structural systems of disadvantage remain firmly in place. Such a reality suggests that future alternative outcomes are precarious at best—or indeed already thwarted. What is at work, then, might be thought of as a perverse ontology: "a turning of the world upside [down] and claiming it is the right side up, it is an interpreted world where the victim becomes the culprit, the violator the aggrieved, the powerful the subaltern."[70]

Regardless of the motivations for medical hot spotting (such as the will to attend to health and affirm life), this biomedical targeting operation actually contradictorily fortifies the cut of race by ontologizing bodies and spaces as a problem, thus reinscribing the epistemology of anti-Blackness. To counter this logic, it becomes imperative to question this epistemology, to work to undo the ways that race functions to biopolitically adjudicate, and to recenter the debt owed to Blacks: by recognizing and actualizing wider social responsibility for conditions of lethality that exclude Blacks (and other minorities) from the possibility of optimal health. To this end, biomedical efforts that seek to organize reparative justice must work against reestablishing race as an ontology at the very same moment that we labor toward alleviating those very real disparities predicated on race.

Such alternative ethical formations and efforts are currently under way in Black Lives Matter organizing and in the practice of medical die-ins (part of the broader Black Lives Matter movement).[71] In response to the chain of preemptive police shootings of unarmed Black subjects in public spaces—and the long historical precedence of coercive force under which Black people have been prefigured as threats in the United States—the multisited Black Lives Matter movement calls out and refuses the foundational epistemology of anti-Blackness that only recognizes and privileges White life and that positions Blacks as a population against which society must be defended. This refusal is enacted through the naming of a project not yet realized: that Black lives matter.[72] The chant calls on people to repudiate the lethal conditions of living out the biopolitical cut of race in America—of no future for Black lives—by asserting what biopolitical futurity has yet to achieve: the so-called universal value that all lives matter.

Medical die-ins or white-coat die-ins counter the perverse ontology we name above. In these events, protestors, usually medical students, lie down motionless, as if dead, on hospital and clinical floors while wearing white coats, the conventional uniform of doctors and a symbol (however problematic) of scientific authority, healing, and responsibility for saving lives. Medical die-ins visually reference and reverse power relations and professional roles within the medical establishment: those who are charged with saving lives paradoxically drop dead. This momentary refusal to be instrumental to pervasive medical institutional racism powerfully draws connections between police brutality against Blacks and the protocols and practices of the U.S. health care system that have led to poorer health, shorter life expectancies, and inferior medical care for Black Americans.[73] The practice marks out the debt owed by those in the medical profession: to take responsibility for previous medical complicity in anti-Blackness and to critically reflect on both the conditions of lethality in neoliberal society and how medicine can (and often does) augment these conditions.

The collective action of suspended medical professional operations—of enacting protest as a professional obligation to public health—opens up the potential to address the role of explicit and implicit forms of discrimination and structural racism in clinical learning environments, medical administrative decision making, medical education curricula, and daily hospital operations. In doing so, white-coat die-ins reject the racialized biopolitics of health because it "kills, sickens, and provides inadequate care."[74] Such enactments ultimately resituate indebtedness away from the vulnerable and disadvantaged and toward a society structured through anti-Blackness. Political action along these lines becomes an ethical imperative in neoliberal times. What remains, however, is the question of how these new ethical formations might translate into practical efforts to redistribute medical care and attention, and how a new sociality might be inaugurated—one that reaffirms civic values and communal interests, and privileges ethical concerns over financial logics.

Notes

1. The practice gained initial national attention in the United States after the publication of a 2011 article: Atul Gawande, "The Hot Spotters," *New Yorker*, January 24, 2011, http://www.newyorker.com/. See also Atul Gawande, "Seeing Spots," *New Yorker*, January 27, 2011, http://www.newyorker.com/. Since then, numerous popular press and medical pieces have been written about the practice, particularly as it has been adopted in other regions of the country and beyond. See, for example, Ryan Meili, who discusses the uptake of the practice in Canada: "How Do We Cool Down Canada's 'Medical Hot Spots'?," *Huffington Post Canada*, November 21, 2013, http://www.huffingtonpost.ca/.

2. On outliers, see Josh Freeman, "Outliers, Hotspotting, and the Social Determinants of Health," *Medicine and Social Justice*, November 23, 2013, http://medicinesocialjustice.blogspot.com.au/. We discuss the conceptualization of certain individuals as socially disintegrated below.

3. Bryce Williams, "Medical Hotspotting: When Treating Patients like Criminals Makes Sense," *Fast Company Co-Exist*, November 23, 2011, http://www.fastcoexist.com/. See also Lisa Duggan, *The Twilight of Equality? Neoliberalism, Cultural Politics, and the Attack on Democracy* (Boston: Beacon Press, 2003); Michael Omi, "'Slippin' into Darkness': The (Re)Biologization of Race," *Journal of Asian American Studies* 13, no. 3 (2010): 343–58.

4. Ruth Wilson Gilmore describes racism as "the state-sanctioned or extra-

legal production and exploitation of group-differentiated vulnerability to premature death." Gilmore, *Golden Gulag: Prisons, Surplus, Crisis, and Opposition in Globalizing California* (Berkeley: University of California Press, 2007), 28.

5. Michel Foucault, *Society Must Be Defended: Lectures at the Collège de France, 1975–1976* (New York: Picador, 2003), 255; Nikolas Rose, *The Politics of Life Itself: Biomedicine, Power, and Subjectivity in the Twenty-First Century* (Princeton, N.J.: Princeton University Press, 2007), 24–25.

6. Michael Dillon and Andrew W. Neal, *Foucault on Politics, Security and War* (London: Palgrave Macmillan, 2008), 168.

7. Such biomedical targeting is evident in the most literal sense in the development of race-specific pharmaceuticals such as BiDil, the first U.S. Food and Drug Administration–approved drug for the treatment of heart failure in self-identified African Americans. See Anne Pollock in this volume. See also Jonathon Kahn, *Race in a Bottle: The Story of BiDil and Racialized Medicine in a Post-genomic Age* (New York: Columbia University Press, 2012); and Anne Pollock, *Medicating Race: Heart Disease and Durable Preoccupations with Difference* (Durham, N.C.: Duke University Press, 2012). Here we move the discussion of biomedical targeting to a wider scale to think about how race is biomedically targeted through health care delivery and practice in medical hot spotting.

8. Anti-Blackness does not "simply name various forms of violence experienced by Blacks, but the violence that *positions* sentient beings outside the realm of the Human." James Bliss, "Hope against Hope: Queer Negativity, Black Feminist Theorizing, and Reproduction Without Futurity," *Mosaic* 48, no. 1 (2015): 89. Frank B. Wilderson considers "the meaning of Blackness not—in the first instance—as a variously and unconsciously interpellated identity or as a conscious social actor [animated by legible political interests], but as a structural position of non-communicability in the face of all other positions." Wilderson, *Red, White, and Black: Cinema and the Structure of U.S. Antagonisms* (Durham, N.C.: Duke University Press, 2010), 58. This positioning stems from liberal humanist thought and is constitutive of Western modernity. See Lindon Barrett, *Racial Blackness and the Discontinuity of Western Modernity*, ed. Justin A. Joyce, Dwight A. McBride, and John Carlos Rowe (Urbana: University of Illinois Press, 2014).

9. Alexander G. Weheliye, *Habeas Viscus: Racializing Assemblages, Biopolitics, and Black Feminist Theories of the Human* (Durham, N.C.: Duke University Press, 2014), 19.

10. For a wide-ranging study, see Harriet A. Washington, *Medical Apartheid: The Dark History of Medical Experimentation on Black Americans from Colonial Times to the Present* (New York: Anchor, 2008). See also Alondra Nelson, *Body and Soul: The Black Panther Party and the Fight against Medical Discrimination* (Minneapolis: University of Minnesota Press, 2011); Dorothy Roberts, *Fatal Invention: How Science, Politics, and Big Business Re-create Race in the*

Twenty-First Century (New York: New Press, 2012); Troy Duster, *Backdoor to Eugenics* (New York: Routledge, 2003); and Michelle van Ryn and Steven S. Fu, "Paved with Good Intentions: Do Public Health and Human Service Providers Contribute to Racial/Ethnic Disparities in Health?," *American Journal of Public Health* 93, no. 2 (2003): 248–55. For reports on racial health disparities, see Brian D. Smedley, Adrienne Y. Smith, and Alan R. Nelson, eds., *Unequal Treatment: Confronting Racial and Ethnic Disparities in Healthcare* (Washington, D.C.: National Academies Press, 2003), https://www.nap.edu/; and the American Medical Association's "Reducing Health Disparities: Where Are We Now?" report, https://www.ama-assn.org/sites/default/files/media-browser/public/public-health/reducing-health-care-disparities-report_1.pdf.

11. W. E. B. Du Bois, *The Philadelphia Negro* (New York: Lippincott, 1899), http://media.pfeiffer.edu/lridener/dss/DuBois/pntoc.html. Henry A. Giroux refers to this as the "biopolitics of disposability," wherein entire populations are marginalized by race and are socially and environmentally excluded from the attainment of health. Giroux, "Reading Hurricane Katrina: Race, Class, and the Biopolitics of Disposability," *College Literature* 33, no. 3 (2006): 171.

12. See Wendy Brown, interviewed by Timothy Shenk, "Booked #3: What Exactly Is Neoliberalism?," *Dissent Magazine*, April 2, 2015, http://www.dissentmagazine.org/.

13. Ibid.

14. See Adele E. Clarke, Janet K. Shim, Laura Mamo, Jennifer Ruth Fosket, and Jennifer R. Fishman, "Biomedicalization: Technoscientific Transformations of Health, Illness, and U.S. Biomedicine," *American Sociological Review* 68, no. 2 (2003): 181–82.

15. On the financialization of health and health care, see Edward J. O'Boyle, "Delivering Health Care in a Financially Broken System," *Personally Speaking*, no. 32 (2007): 1–5, http://www.mayoresearch.org/files/FINANCIALIZATION32.pdf.

16. On pastoral power, see Michel Foucault, *Security, Territory, Population: Lectures at the Collège de France, 1977–78*, ed. Michel Senellart, trans. Graham Burchell (London: Palgrave MacMillan, 2007), 126–29.

17. Nancy Leong, "Racial Capitalism," *Harvard Law Review* 126, no. 8 (2013): 2151–226.

18. Henry A. Giroux, "Spectacles of Race and Pedagogies of Denial: Anti-Black Racist Pedagogy under the Reign of Neoliberalism," *Communication Education* 52, no. 3/4 (2003): 195–96.

19. Medical hot spotting developed in response to Camden's extensive violence and medical indigence experienced by its mostly African American and Latino population. Just as hot spotting has been generalized and put to work in a variety of locations, the historical geography of Camden is also both specific and generalizable—perhaps an extreme version of conditions experienced in many other parts of the United States.

20. See "Quick Facts: Camden City, New Jersey," *United States Census Bureau,* http://www.census.gov/.
21. Figure from CamConnect's 2008 "Camden Facts," http://www.camconnect.org/datalogue/Camden_Facts_08_3-20-08_health.pdf.
22. Jianying Hu, Fei Wang, Jimeng Sun, Robert Sorrentino, and Shahram Ebadollahi, "A Healthcare Utilization Analysis Framework for Hot Spotting and Contextual Anomaly Detection," *American Medical Informatics Association Annual Symposium Proceedings* (2012): 360–69.
23. Dylan Ratigan, "Hot-Spotting: It's How, Not How Much," *Dylan Ratigan* (blog), November 28, 2011, http://www.dylanratigan.com/.
24. There are numerous short biographies of Brenner and popular accounts of the development of medical hot spotting; see Gawande, "Hot Spotters." Brenner was a medical student at Robert Wood Johnson Medical School and on track to becoming a neuroscientist when he volunteered at a free primary care clinic for poor immigrants and changed his mind. He completed his residency and joined a family medicine practice in Camden.
25. Williams, "Medical Hotspotting."
26. While rudimentary human compiling and handmade maps can serve to locate problem areas and populations, the goal is ultimately to integrate advanced machine learning techniques into a care management application that can perform systematic analysis on any given patient population in order to identify cases of high utilization. See Hu et al., "Healthcare Utilization Analysis Framework," 361.
27. Dr. Jeffrey C. Brenner, "Finding Hot Spots: A How-To Interview with Jeffrey Brenner," interview by Carol Peckham, *Medscape,* June 6, 2012, http://www.medscape.com/.
28. Brenner's figures are from "How 'Hot Spotting' Cut Health Care Costs by 50%," *Robert Wood Johnson Foundation,* http://www.rwjf.org/ (no longer available online).
29. Peter Bronski, "The Doctor on a Medical Mission," *Vassar: The Alumnae/i Quarterly* 108, no. 2 (2012), http://vq.vassar.edu/.
30. Ibid.
31. Haydn Bush, "Health Care's Costliest 1%," *Hospitals and Health Networks,* September 1, 2012, http://www.hhnmag.com/.
32. Bronski, "Doctor on a Medical Mission."
33. Brenner has also emphasized the importance of garnering qualitative data from doctors and providers in the process of locating high utilizers.
34. "Aetna Foundation Awards $325,000 in Grants to Train Doctors for 21st-Century Health Care," press release, *Aetna Foundation,* March 5, 2013, http://news.aetnafoundation.org/.
35. The Patient Protection and Affordable Care Act (PPACA) was signed into law on March 2010; it will reportedly spend $848 billion through 2020 on health

reform. See Brenner, "Finding Hot Spots"; John Blair, "Universal Hot Spotting: The Future of American Medicine in the Face of a Novel Healthcare Delivery Approach," *Triple Helix,* http://asutriplehelix.org/node/185 (no longer available online).

36. Brenner, "Finding Hot Spots."

37. See Gawande, "Seeing Spots" and "Hot Spotters." Other pilot programs of patient-focused accountable care include the Special Care Program in Seattle for Boeing workers; CareOregon's geomapping of high-cost users as part of its administration of a nonprofit health plan that serves Medicare and Medicaid patients; and Southcentral Foundation's health care system in Anchorage, Alaska, which targets Native Alaskans to coordinate care and cut costs. It is important to note that when we were initially researching medical hot spotting, the practice was just beginning. At that time, it was largely community based and focused on individuals. Since then, it has spread and moved into institutions, and it has become heavily bureaucratized.

38. The institutional racism of medicine includes lack of economic access to health care in relation to racial stratification of the economy; barriers to hospitals and health care institutions resulting from the closure, relocation, or privatization of hospitals that primarily serve minority populations; inequities in preventive care and treatment based on medical or biological differences, income, and so on; lack of culturally competent care and/or language accessibility; racial disparities in the provision of treatments and inclusion in research; unequal access to emergency care and excessive wait times; deposit requirements as a prerequisite to care; and the refusal of Medicaid patients. An extended review is provided in Vernellia Randall, "Institutional Racism in U.S. Health Care," *Institute on Race, Health Care, and the Law,* n.d., http://academic.udayton.edu/. See also David G. Whiteis, "Unhealthy Cities: Corporate Medicine, Community Economic Underdevelopment, and Public Health," *International Journal of Health Services* 27, no. 2 (1997): 227–42, esp. 227.

39. Jenna Loyd, *Health Rights Are Civil Rights: Peace and Justice Activism in Los Angeles, 1963–1978* (Minneapolis: University of Minnesota Press, 2014), 30.

40. George Lipsitz incisively observes, "Competition for scarce resources in the North American context generates new racial enmities and antagonisms, which in turn promotes new variants of racism." Lipsitz, *American Studies in a Moment of Danger* (Minneapolis: University of Minnesota Press, 2001), 12.

41. Whiteis sounded an early warning in the late 1990s: "The current emphasis on 'managing' medical care for cost containment disregards the social and environmental genesis of many health problems." Whiteis, "Unhealthy Cities," 229.

42. Doug Eby, MD, vice president of medical services for Southcentral Foundation health care system, Anchorage, Alaska, quoted in Bush, "Health Care's Costliest 1%"; Ed Sealover, "'Hot Spotting' May Be Way to Cool Cost of Health Care," *Denver Business Journal,* July 27, 2012, http://www.bizjournals.com/.

43. "Uncompensated Hospital Care Cost Fact Sheet," *American Hospital Association,* January 2014, http://www.acainternational.org/. Importantly, uncompensated care debt excludes other unfunded costs of care, such as underpayment from Medicaid and Medicare.

44. See "The Uninsured: Access to Medical Care," news release, *American College of Emergency Physicians,* n.d., http://www.acep.org/; *American Hospital Association,* January 2016 "Uncompensated Hospital Care Cost Fact Sheet," http://www.aha.org/content/16/uncompensatedcarefactsheet.pdf. At the time of this chapter's writing, figures were not yet available for 2013–14.

45. April Michelle Herndon, "Collateral Damage from Friendly Fire? Race, Nation, Class and the 'War against Obesity,'" *Social Semiotics* 15, no. 2 (2005): 132.

46. Raj Bhopal, "Spectre of Racism in Health and Health Care: Lessons from History and the United States," *BMJ* 316, no. 7149 (1998): 1970–73.

47. Whiteis, "Unhealthy Cities," 229.

48. David J. Roberts and Minelle Mahtani, "Neoliberalizing Race, Racing Neoliberalism: Placing 'Race' in Neoliberal Discourses," *Antipode* 42, no. 2 (2010): 249. Roberts and Mahtani are paraphrasing the arguments of David Wilson, *Cities and Race: America's New Black Ghettos* (New York: Routledge, 2006).

49. Elizabeth Povinelli, "The Child in the Broom Closet," *States of Violence: War, Capital Punishment, and Letting Die,* ed. Austin Sarat and Jennifer L. Culbert (Cambridge: Cambridge University Press, 2009), 177.

50. Institute of Medicine of the National Academy, Committee on the Consequences of Uninsurance, Board on Health Care Services, *Hidden Costs, Values Lost: Uninsurance in America* (Washington, D.C.: National Academies Press, 2003).

51. Dana-Ain Davis, "Narrating the Mute: Racializing and Racism in a Neoliberal Moment," *Souls* 9, no. 4 (2007): 349.

52. Bush, "Health Care's Costliest 1%," 32.

53. See, for example, the *Frontline* video "Doctor Hotspot," *PBS,* July 26, 2011, http://video.pbs.org/video/2070853636/.

54. Loïc Wacquant forcefully argues that welfare and penal policies are linked, "inasmuch as these two strands of government action toward the poor have come to be informed by the same behaviorist philosophy relying on deterrence, surveillance, stigma, and graduated sanctions to modify conduct." Wacquant, "Crafting the Neoliberal State: Workfare, Prisonfare, and Social Insecurity," *Sociological Forum* 25, no. 2 (2010): 199.

55. Torin Monahan and Tyler Wall, "Somatic Surveillance: Corporeal Control through Information Networks," *Surveillance and Society* 4, no. 3 (2007): 163; Herndon, "Collateral Damage," 132.

56. Amy Finkelstein, Ruohua Annetta Zhou, Sarah Taubman, Joseph Doyle, and Jeffrey Brenner, "Health Care Hotspotting: A Randomized Controlled Trial Analysis Plan," study AEARCTR-0000329, *American Economic Association Randomized Controlled Trial Registry,* March 7, 2014, https://www.socialscienceregistry.org/;

see also "Health Care Hotspotting: A Randomized Controlled Trial," study NCT02090426, *Smart Patients,* https://www.smartpatients.com/.

57. Wacquant, "Crafting the Neoliberal State," 218.

58. Generally speaking, workfare is a punitive system whereby individuals must work or attempt to secure work—and submit themselves to rigorous auditing processes—in order to continue to qualify for welfare aid.

59. George L. Kelling and William J. Bratton, "Declining Crime Rates: Insiders' Views of the New York City Story," *Journal of Criminal Law and Criminology* 88, no. 4 (1998): 1217–31; Amy Propen, "Critical GPS: Toward a New Politics of Location," *ACME* 4, no. 1 (2006): 135. Bratton was the New York City police commissioner twice, leaving his second stint in 2016.

60. Williams, "Medical Hotspotting."

61. Whether for biosecurity or target marketing purposes, spatial profiling measures and maps, and in doing so, it sets up the possibility of expectations that can be linked to spaces and populations through the act of targeting. Targeting territorializes such expectations and involves place-particularizing metaphors, masculinist ideas about penetrating and mastering space, and a network logic (i.e., targets are under the purview of a larger, more encompassing gaze and database). Targeting in terms of "seeing as destroying" is beyond the scope here.

62. Targeting promises powerful technological mastery by the long-standing martial and territorial aspects of mapping combined with the virtualizing of the world through technology as information. See Stephen Graham, *Cities Under Siege: The New Military Urbanism* (London: Verso, 2011), xi; Matthew Sparke, "From Global Dispossession to Local Repossession: Towards a Worldly Cultural Geography of Occupy Activism," in *The New Companion to Cultural Geography,* ed. Huala Johnson, Richard Schein, and Jamie Winders (Oxford: Wiley-Blackwell, 2013), 387–408; Jeremy W. Crampton, "The Biopolitical Justification for Geosurveillance," *Geographical Review* 97, no. 3 (2007): 389–90; Derek Gregory, "'In Another Time-Zone, the Bombs Fall Unsafely . . .': Targets, Civilians and Late Modern War," July 2012, http://geographicalimaginations.files.wordpress.com/2012/07/gregory-in-another-time-zone_illustrated.pdf; Rey Chow, *The Age of the World Target: Self-Referentiality in War, Theory, and Comparative Work* (Durham, N.C.: Duke University Press, 2006), 40; Caren Kaplan, "Precision Targets: GPS and the Militarization of U.S. Consumer Identity," *American Quarterly* 58, no. 3 (2006): 693–713, esp. 694–95; Samuel Weber, *Targets of Opportunity: On the Militarization of Thinking* (New York: Fordham University, 2005).

63. Kaplan, "Precision Targets," 697.

64. Racialized spaces and bodies become ontologized in space as locationally removed, knowable, and measurable data of a population, which in essence normalizes racism as just another map of everyday life. Accordingly, medical hot spots might be seen to ontologize the ghetto, reinforcing and further entrenching

existing racialized segregations, including the historical geographies of urban renewal, redlining in housing and mortgage industries, and environmental racism.

65. Propen, "Critical GPS," 136.

66. Wacquant, "Crafting the Neoliberal State"; Loïc Wacquant, "From Slavery to Mass Incarceration: Rethinking the 'Race Question' in the U.S.," *New Left Review* 13 (2002): 41–60.

67. Graham, *Cities Under Siege*, 99.

68. Katharyne Mitchell, "Pre-Black Futures," *Antipode* 41, no. 1 (2009): 239–61, 254. Part of the legacy of militarized visual culture, the targeting operations of medical hot spotting dramatically translate military dreams of high-tech omniscience and rationality into the governance of urban civil society, extending the military-industrial complex into everyday life to govern race as biosecurity threat.

69. Through the lens of anti-Black epistemology, Black subjects could be understood as posing a threat to the health of the population as a whole in that their ill health (which, as we argue, is produced through a whole series of past and present social factors) introduces disequilibrium into the population. Rather than addressing the social causes of ill health, however, Blacks are blamed as the cause of this disequilibrium.

70. Amareswar Galla and Conrad Gershevitch, "Freedom of Religion and Belief, Culture, and the Arts: A Supplementary Paper Prepared for the Australian Human Rights Commission and the Australia Council for the Arts to Complement the Research Report," *Australian Human Rights Commission*, 2010, https://www.humanrights.gov.au/sites/default/files/content/frb/papers/FRB%20arts.pdf.

71. Another direction we could have taken in thinking through the politics of refusal would have been to look at the important place of health in historical struggles for social change and historical social movements against anti-Black violence; see, for example, Loyd, *Health Rights Are Civil Rights*.

72. Judith Butler, interviewed by George Yancy, "What's Wrong with 'All Lives Matter'?," *New York Times*, January 12, 2015, http://opinionator.blogs.nytimes.com/.

73. Renee Lewis, "Medical Students Stage Nationwide Die-in over Racial Bias in Health Care," *Aljazeera America*, December 10, 2014, http://america.aljazeera.com/.

74. "Medical Students to Hold Nationwide 'Die-ins' and Protests Wednesday Because #BlackLivesMatter," press release, *Physicians for National Health Program*, December 9, 2014, http://www.pnhp.org/.

3

Obamacare and Sovereign Debt
Race, Reparations, and the Haunting of Premature Death

JENNA M. LOYD

> The pillars of American liberalism—the Democratic Party, the universities and the mass media—are obsessed with biological markers, most particularly race and gender. They have insisted, moreover, that pedagogy and culture and politics be just as seized with the primacy of these distinctions and with the resulting "privileging" that allegedly haunts every aspect of our social relations.
> —CHARLES KRAUTHAMMER, "ADVENTURES IN IDENTITY POLITICS" (2008)

> Race-based medicine helps promote a biological explanation for racial inequities that obscures their sociopolitical causes and requires individualized and market-based solutions rather than social change. By making black people's subordinated status seem natural, this view provides a ready logic for the staggering disenfranchisement of black citizens, as well as the perfect complement to colorblind social policies.
> —DOROTHY ROBERTS, "IS RACE-BASED MEDICINE GOOD FOR US?" (2008)

American racial politics during the age of President Barack Obama has been haunted, though perhaps not in the ways meant by Charles Krauthammer. During the 2008 Democratic Party primary battle between Hillary Clinton and Barack Obama, Krauthammer, the "sober elder statesman among today's conservative commentariat," observed that "biological markers, particularly of race and gender" had grown into a "full flowering of identity politics."[1] Not optimistic that the "looming ugly endgame" would soon end, he offered that his fellow "pessimist will vote Republican."[2]

Krauthammer hints at the social construction of race and gender by using the term "privilege," but he then reinscribes identity to biology. Krauthammer's remarks tacitly invoke the ostensible biological differences between a (white) woman's and (Black, biracial) man's bodies to claim for conservatives the moral high road of meritocracy through blindness to "color" and gender.[3] That is, he simultaneously appropriates for the Republicans the long-standing rejection of biology as the basis for drawing social distinctions while continuing to conflate social difference with biology, a rhetorical move that renders liberal identity politics as fatuous and time bound.[4]

Until, that is, the GOP was in the midst of its own internecine battle over sovereign debt and medicine, in which race and identity politics were always present and made absent. On August 21, 2013, newly elected congressman Mark Meadows (R-NC) delivered a letter signed by seventy-nine other House Republicans to John Boehner, then the Speaker of the House, and Eric Cantor, the House majority leader. The aim of their appeal was to "affirmatively de-fund the implementation and enforcement of ObamaCare in any relevant appropriations bill brought to the House floor in the 113th Congress, including any continuing appropriations bill."

Their grievance? The imminent rollout of the Patient Protection and Affordable Care Act (ACA), the most comprehensive reform of American health care policy since the passage of Medicare and Medicaid in 1965. Many Republicans, like Meadows, had made repealing the legislation a major part of their campaign strategy during the 2010 midterm elections. Backed by the libertarian FreedomWorks organization and populist Tea Party protests, they made huge gains in the House of Representatives and at the state level. Among the reasons for their opposition was the claim that the health reform would destroy the American economy. Boehner, in his first speech as Speaker of the House, reiterated their message, though he was not in favor of the shutdown: "It will ruin the best health care system in the world. It will bankrupt our nation, and it will ruin our economy!"[5]

Despite picking up over sixty seats to take over the House, and over thirty attempts to repeal the ACA between January 2011 and fall 2012, the GOP remained unsuccessful because Democrats continued to hold the Senate.[6] This group of Republicans, whom Krauthammer would soon dub the "suicide caucus," thus sought Boehner's help in using Congress's power to authorize additional federal debt to prevent the implementation of the ACA. Refusing to issue new debt would mean that the federal government would not have money to fund its operations, save for defense. To bolster the righteousness of their action, the group invoked James Madison's observation in the *Federalist Papers* that "the power of the purse may, in fact, be regarded as the most complete and effectual weapon . . . for obtaining a redress of every grievance."[7]

Here I focus on this moment of conflict over the ACA to explore how the threat of default on the sovereign debt was leveraged on and against Black and poor people's bodies. Deploying the purse as a weapon—and the violence of this tactic is explicitly stated—to halt the ACA also had near immediate effects on programs on which low-income people survive, such as Head Start early childhood education and vouchers for the Special Supplemental Nutrition Program for Women, Infants, and Children, and threatened others.[8] For decades, Republicans discursively have been connecting entitlement programs to sovereign indebtedness, depicting poor people's lives in net negative terms. The ideological work of such biopolitical leveraging displaces the far more significant contributions that tax cuts and spending in other sectors of the budget, such as defense, make to national spending and debt.[9]

Perhaps the most important discussion to be hijacked during the 2013 government shutdown was the relationship between universal health care and the past and present harms of structural racism. The bodily materiality of such racism marked by heightened rates of Black morbidity and premature death—past and present—remained submerged, disavowed, unspeakable. Quantifying such health harms has not been a neutral practice; it has been a political project of conceptualization and categorization. I situate the debate over Obamacare within a longer history of reforms over the past six decades that have unevenly (by geography, class, race, and citizenship status) expanded access to health care. Even as millions more Americans have gained greater access to health care—and have thereby been drawn into expanding circuits and flows of capital in the health sector—there have always been exclusions. These exclusions have tracked interlocking lines of race and class, concentrating rather than ameliorating suffering and premature deaths in Black and poor communities. In turn, race-based medicine (and public health interventions) have often been designed to target remedies on bodies as racial objects. Yet, following Dorothy Roberts's contention in the epigraph, such strategies work to naturalize the social, economic, and political processes that produce racialized suffering and death.

The struggle over the ACA is an example of race-based medicine at the level of access to and dignified care within the health care system. I analyze this conflict not because access to health care is the only or most significant determinant of health or longevity; the vast literature on the social and structural determinants of health illustrates that redistribution of wealth and investments in equitable affordable housing and education, job creation, a guaranteed annual income, and ending reliance on imprisonment would be significant health-promoting policies.[10] I am interested in how efforts to block expanded access to health care under the ACA explicitly perpetuate existing social and health injustices, and thereby sanction premature deaths. Struggles over access to health care as a racial (biopolitical) line expose how value circulates within the body politic, thus dividing the worthy and unworthy along racial and class lines, and how some people's premature deaths can accumulate for others as wealth, health, and political power.

Sovereign Debt, Race, and the Suicide Caucus

The gambit by Mark Meadows, Ted Cruz, and fellow Tea Party Republicans to block implementation of the ACA in 2013 involved a combination of legislative moves, including refusing to increase the federal debt ceiling and appropriations for federal government operations. The timing of their move was essential. In early 2012, the chairman of the Federal Reserve, Ben Bernanke, began issuing warnings about the dangers of the looming fiscal cliff—the confluence of tax increases (including the expiration of Bush-era tax cuts) and spending cuts (sequestration) that would result from the failure to pass a deficit reduction deal—which would transpire in January 2013. The presidential election and differing analyses on the consequences of this fiscal free fall, including debates over who would be most harmed by cuts to entitlement and regulatory programs that many Republicans wanted to starve, were part of the impasse over 2012 budget negotiations. Going over the fiscal cliff would result in a sharp decrease in sovereign debt, but as *CNN Money* warned, "because it would be so abrupt and arbitrary, it also could throw the United States back into a recession next year, when more than $500 billion will be taken out of the economy."[11]

By 2013, threatening to shut down the government as a tactic to abolish the ACA struck commentators from across the political spectrum (and many corporate leaders) as dangerously misguided. Krauthammer told *Inside Washington* that he "admire[s] the sincerity and the passion of those who don't want to pass the budget unless you get rid of Obamacare."[12] He warned, however, that their efforts "would be over a cliff for the GOP."[13] Their tactics were so wrong-headed that they had effectively joined a suicide caucus, a direct retort to Texas senator Ted Cruz, who had derided Republicans opposed to the defunding tactic by calling them a "surrender caucus."[14] Despite sharp criticism from fellow Republicans, these eighty members of the House moved forward and blocked the passage of a compromise appropriations bill to fund government operations beginning on October 1, 2013.

For the next several weeks, as the federal government was partially shuttered, the suicide caucus circulated as a frame to discuss crises in the Republican Party and the United States' representative democracy. While conservative critics were concerned that this tactic threatened the future of the GOP, both conservative and liberal pundits were concerned about the implications that this minority bloc's actions posed to U.S. global power. China's official Xinhua news agency wrote that the shutdown illustrated "the ugly side of partisan politics in Washington."[15] Indeed, President Obama canceled his trip to the Asia Pacific Economic Cooperation summit, and commentators worried that the "current situation in the United States has created a disaster for U.S. foreign policy in the Asia-Pacific region. And you can be sure that China will be there, making hay."[16]

Commentators invoked historical political geographies to make sense of how race informed contemporary political patterns. *New Yorker* commentator Ryan Lizza noted that "half of these [suicide caucus] districts are concentrated in the South, and a quarter of them are in the Midwest."[17] "Naturally," he continued, "there are no members from New England, the megalopolis corridor from Washington to Boston, or along the Pacific coastline."[18] Implicit within his analysis is that sectional disputes over slavery, Jim Crow, and race continue to weigh on contemporary politics. The *New York Times* backed this narrative with a lead story accompanied by interactive maps detailing who would be left out of the ACA. The section of the ACA stipulating that states would extend coverage through their Medicaid programs had been struck down by the Supreme Court in 2012 in *National Federation of Independent Business v. Sebelius*. This ruling meant that poor Americans living in one of twenty-six states that were not extending Medicaid would be left out of the ACA. About half of all Americans lived in these states, but almost 70 percent of poor uninsured Black people lived here.[19] To underscore the significance of this ruling, the *Times* turned to medical doctor, community health advocate, and civil rights activist H. Jack Geiger, who observed: "The irony is that these states that are rejecting Medicaid expansion—many of them Southern—are the very places where the concentration of poverty and lack of health insurance are the most acute."[20]

Yet Southern exceptionalism and history alone could not explain the Tea Party bloc, or where Medicaid was not expanded. Lizza reminds readers of contemporary racial dynamics, observing, "Members of the suicide caucus live in a different America from the one that most political commentators describe when talking about how the country is transforming. The average suicide-caucus district is seventy-five per cent white, while the average House district is sixty-three per cent white."[21] While rates of health insurance were almost identical across congressional districts represented by Republicans and Democrats (14.1 to 15.6 percent uninsured), the ideological import of the ACA "trump[ed] interest for Republicans."[22] Largely forgotten were the conservative, market-based origins of the program—mandates requiring the purchase of insurance and health insurance exchanges—which formed the basis of the Massachusetts universal insurance model implemented while Republican Mitt Romney was governor of that state.[23]

Rather, there was a fraught conversation about race undertaken within the terms of color-blindness and what David Theo Goldberg terms racial neoliberalism. If we conceive of capitalism as always ever racial capitalism and the state in the United States as a racial state, contemporary capitalist and state restructuring necessarily rework racial relations.[24] Many use the term "neoliberalism" to describe systemic shifts in capitalism and the state since the early 1970s, which have involved often debt-induced pressure to deregulate trade, industry, and environmental, health, and labor protections; privatize state industries and services; and reduce government spending on social services.[25] Within the context of racial neoliberalism, Goldberg argues that racism is unmoored from historical roots and is individualized. Discursively, the racial is severed from the sphere of politics and the public domain and "restrict[ed] to the privacy of occasional individual choice and (self-)determination. [. . .] Race is rendered accordingly before, beneath, or beyond the law."[26] The problem of racism becomes "*invoking* race, not [. . .] its debilitating structural effects or the legacy of its ongoing unfair impacts."[27]

Indeed, some took pains to distance their opposition to the ACA from charges of racism. MSNBC host and former Republican congressman Joe Scarborough remarked:

> I must say, I have been behind closed doors with thousands of conservatives through the years. I have never once heard one of them say in

the deep south or in the northeast or in South Boston, "Boy, I really hate Obamacare because that black president"—no, I've never heard anybody come close to saying that.[28]

Defining racism narrowly as an attribute of individual statements and stereotypically racist places enables Scarborough to refute racism because he had not heard people utter transparently racist words. Conservative talk show host Rush Limbaugh did explicitly invoke race through the specter of Black power. For him, the ACA "is a civil rights bill, this is reparations, whatever you want to call it," and he suggested that Obama "just wants us to have the same health care plan that he had in Kenya."[29] His invocation of Kenya trades in both the racist birther conspiracy theory (which claims that Obama was not born in the United States and therefore is ineligible for the presidency) and in the imagination of Kenya as inferior to the United States.

Bill O'Reilly, like Limbaugh, bristled at the idea that policies could be crafted to resolve historical injustice: "I think Mr. Obama allows historical grievances—things like slavery, bad treatment for Native Americans and U.S. exploitation of Third World countries—to shape his economic thinking.... He gives the bad things about America far too much weight, leading to his desire to redistribute wealth, thereby correcting historical grievance."[30] The history that Limbaugh and O'Reilly invoke is a past that is past, and for which wrongs have been righted. The conceit that people of color seek revenge amplifies their characterization of the ACA as unjust given their position that the nation is not today structured by past "bad things" that would require healing and redistribution. Yet within the logic of racial neoliberalism, inequities by definition cannot exist. Thus, marshaling evidence of a systematically produced inequity becomes evidence for "unfair" race consciousness and for opposing a policy that would partially remedy inequitable health care access.

Given that states are not obliged to expand their Medicaid programs to those who are eligible (which is also variable across states), the ACA has not remedied racialized and class-based exclusion from health care or histories of exploitation within medicine.[31] Indeed, health care alone cannot remedy what physicians W. Michael Byrd and Linda A. Clayton refer to as the "slave health deficit"—that is, health inequities rooted in chattel slavery and perpetuated by institutionalized racism in medicine and other institutions.[32] Reparations as a way of reckoning with and acknowledging social injury links backward- and forward-looking temporalities to inform social and political transformation of injustices rooted in those harms.[33] Reparations, conceived of as debts that are owed, raises questions not only of repayment (and in what material and moral terms) but also of how social and economic value circulates within the social body. How does the redress for harms that Meadows's letter invoked to block the ACA circulate in relation to the erasure of white supremacy and the color-blind claim that U.S. society has been racially reconciled? Given that premature deaths are a result of structural violence, how can repayment or restitution be made for these prematurely shortened lives?

Haunting and the Embodied Circuits of Debt and Premature Death

I turn to Lauren Berlant's work on slow death and Avery Gordon's work on haunting to analyze how temporality, value, and death figure in debates over the ACA. Berlant introduces the term "slow death" to conceptualize shifts in politics and agency in the context of contemporary capitalism. The dismantling of the social wage and futurity of a "better life" once expected by many Americans has entailed the "attrition of the subject" and a reconstitution of relations between accretive (life-building) activities and more pragmatic, everyday activities. Health is one realm where such subjective shifts can be discerned because it has so long served as a marker of appropriate life-extending subjectivity. Markers of healthy eating, sexual responsibility, and riskiness index social norms and difference in ways that enable "political crises to be cast as conditions of specific bodies and their competence at maintaining health or other conditions of social belonging."[34]

For Berlant, such frames of crisis hold limited political promise for the left because "slow death—or the structurally induced attrition of persons keyed to their membership in certain populations—is neither a state of exception nor the opposite, mere banality, but a domain where the upsetting scene of living is revealed to be interwoven with the ordinary life after all."[35] By way of example, Berlant analyzes the contemporary obesity crisis, which dominant health and political discourses narrate as one of excessive individual sovereignty (or agency). Thus, the invocation of crisis works to shore up a diminishing notion of the subject even as it obscures "long-term problems of embodiment within capitalism, in the zoning of the everyday, the work of getting through it, and the obstacles to physical and mental flourishing."[36]

Circuits of capital that flow through and differentially accumulate in landscapes and bodies simultaneously work as a "disintegrating circuit."[37] For Berlant, material wealth, health, and political power accumulate systematically through processes that result in the deterioration, attrition, and disintegration of the bodies of working-class and marginalized groups of people. While these disintegrated bodies may only sometimes generate capital through performing labor, Berlant argues that representing them as sites of nonvalue or negative value is false. Not only do they remain profitably integrated into capitalist food—and, I would add, health care—markets, but also negative representations of overweight people as failed subjects are valuable figures within capitalist circuits of distributing value. "Healthy living" and appropriate consumption of health care have long served as criteria for distinguishing worthy and unworthy subjects and for directing resources into respective circuits of social investment or disintegration and abandonment.[38]

Over 42 million people were uninsured before the passage of the ACA, which made payment for debt a central framing of the policy problem. Supreme Court justice Ruth Bader Ginsberg's dissenting opinion on *National Federation of Independent Business v. Sebelius* observes: "Health-care providers do not absorb these bad debts [for unpaid care for the uninsured]. Instead, they raise their prices, passing along the cost of uncompensated care to those who do pay reliably: the government and private insurance companies."[39] In neoclassical economic terms, this group is framed as free riders. People without health insurance become a threat to the insured and to the broader health care system because of their failure to function as paying bodies in a circuit of services, exchange, and accumulation. In this logic, insolvency is spread across the social body in ways that threaten corporate profit and national competitiveness. The expansion of the ACA, then, is a moment in the restructuring of the racial state wherein social deservingness is marked through marketability. Meanwhile, the principle of health rights based in mutual obligation, the debts we owe each other, is effectively devalued.

Berlant uses the temporality of slowness to describe the protracted, everyday embodiment of exploitation and attrition. The uninsured as a social category perhaps best exemplify the condition of slow death, with some 45,000 people dying in the United States annually as a result of lack of insurance.[40] What happens to disintegrating bodies after they have been rendered a social sacrifice? Do they disappear? How do we understand the acceleration of slow deaths, such as with the recent sharp uptick in mortality among middle-aged white people?[41] How can we understand slow deaths in relation to the abrupt deaths of the 400 people whom the police annually kill in acts classified as "justifiable homicide"?[42] Can they, and the deaths from public policy exclusion, be accounted for alongside those of Oscar Grant, Trayvon Martin, Michael Brown, Chantel Davis, and other people, principally Black and Brown, killed by the police and vigilantes? How—or, more accurately, for whom—is the accumulation of premature deaths through a potent mix of daily, grinding structural violence and punctuated, though systemic, acts of state aggression not a crisis?

Avery Gordon's concept of haunting can help answer these questions. Simply, these slow and fast and premature and excess deaths are with us. "They produce material effects" within and beyond capitalist circuits.[43] "The ghost," Gordon writes, "is not simply a dead or missing person, but a social figure, and investigating it can lead to that dense site where history and subjectivity make social life."[44] Where Krauthammer's invocation of haunting and Limbaugh's framing of the ACA as reparations attempt to partition the past from present, the haunting that I observe in the debate over the ACA is the exploitation of premature deaths to further accumulate wealth and entrench racial state power.

Racism, following Ruth Wilson Gilmore, is "state-sanctioned and or extra legal production and exploitation of group-differentiated vulnerabilities to premature death."[45] This definition registers the materiality and relationality of racism, with the term "production" registering the creation of harmful social and economic conditions and the term "exploitation" indexing the power and resources that dominant groups accumulate from such deadly conditions. Thus, in considering the value of repair, or debts owed for unjustly shortened lives, one place to begin is in recognizing that these lives do not disappear. Rather, they haunt the present, and the conditions responsible for their unjust deaths continue to undergird contemporary social and economic life.

Gilmore's definition of racism can be understood within a long history of critical temporalities and categories developed for counting and countering the material toll of racism and structural violence. W. E. B. Du Bois used the concept of excess death to challenge racist claims that higher rates of Black mortality were a result of bodily inferiority. By documenting the increase of mortality rates over time and variability across Northern and Southern cities, he showed that "the matter of sickness is an indication of social and economic position" not biology.[46] Du Bois observed, moreover, that, "the amount paid for sickness is highest among the poorer classes and lowest among the better-to-do. It seems that the sickness bill increases inversely with wages."[47] Several decades later, medical doctor M. Alfred Haynes likened the gap between white and Black life expectancy to a historical disjuncture wherein Black people could expect lives to extend to "the level of the White population of about

30 years ago."[48] Each of these concepts offers a way for recognizing the bodily harms—in shortened lives, missing people, and blocked human progress—that result from racial domination.

As the introduction to this book details, health researchers have continued to document the fact that health inequalities track racial and socioeconomic inequalities. The publication of a multivolume report on white–Black health disparities by the Department of Health and Human Services found that 47 percent of all deaths of Black men and women under the age of forty-five were excessive, as were 42 percent of deaths of Black men and women under the age of seventy.[49] This report placed racial health disparities on the U.S. policy agenda, informing the objectives of Healthy People 2000 to reduce health inequities.[50]

After the gains of the 1965–75 "'civil rights era' in health care" for African Americans, Byrd and Clayton ruefully concluded that the "commitment, political support, and funding for these stopgap measures waned, [and] blacks' progress in health stopped by 1975."[51] Reversals in Black mortality in the 1980s challenged presumptions of (biomedical) progress and drew renewed attention to the importance of social and structural determinants of health, including the role that investments in living conditions and minimum incomes play in ameliorating structural racism.

Between 1980 and 2000, standardized mortality rates for African Americans remained essentially the same or were slightly higher, while there was an overall decline for white Americans.[52] This widening gap is disconcerting in its own right, but it masks sharp temporal and geographical variation. In the 1980s, there was an increase in death rates for young people (aged fifteen to twenty-four; twenty-five to thirty-four; and thirty-five to forty-four) principally due to AIDS, homicide, and suicide.[53] Between 1983 and 1988, Joseph Mangano calculated that this reversal resulted in nearly 14,000 excess deaths.[54] Among Black people in these age groups, death rates not due to AIDS increased 23.4, 6.0, and 7.6 percent, respectively—figures he called "nothing short of shocking."[55] In short, young Black people living in high-poverty urban areas could expect worse mortality rates into middle age in 1990 compared to 1980.[56]

Significant decreases in homicides contributed to declines in mortality between 1990 and 2000, but decreases in excess deaths due to circulatory disease or cancer were not as significant.[57] For people living in rural areas, absolute death rates among women actually worsened between 1980 and 2000, as did excess death rates and standardized mortality rates among men and women.[58] These findings led Arline Geronimus and colleagues to conclude that "failure to adequately address excessive rates of chronic disease in high-poverty locales limited the extent to which progress was made in reducing excess mortality in vulnerable populations" and attributed this failing to higher rates of disease prevalence and lack of adequate health care.[59]

Histories of Class and Racial Exclusion in Health Care Reform

Equitable health care is one element of a broader project of ending racial capitalism. While only 10 to 15 percent of preventable deaths in the United States can be attributed to medical care, uneven access to dignified health care contributes to racial, class, and gender inequities in quality of life and longevity.[60] Nearly twenty years after the Department of Health and Human Services report on racial health disparities, George W. Bush administration officials ordered researchers to strike the use of the term in the Institute of Medicine's 562-page report *Unequal Treatment*.[61] The uncensored report was released under pressure from congressional Democrats; it found that "evidence of racial and ethnic disparities in healthcare is, with few exceptions, remarkably consistent across a range of illnesses and healthcare services," including racial disparities in screening for cancer and treatment, quality of HIV care, and cardiovascular care that result in higher mortality rates or poorer survival rates among people of color.[62] H. Jack Geiger's review chapter of 600 published studies on racial/ethnic disparities in health care diagnosis and treatment concluded, "Among the multiple causes of racial and ethnic disparities in American health care, provider and institutional bias are significant contributors."[63] Moreover, "compared with those deeply entrenched causes [inequitable social and physical environments], provider and institutional bias are far more directly (though not easily) remediable, and represent an opportunity for rapid change."[64]

Even though universal health care alone cannot resolve the racial inequities within the health care system, failure to extend access to health care, such as through Medicaid, exacerbates the problem. Evidence from the Oregon Health Insurance Experiment found that after being enrolled in Medicaid for seventeen months, people experienced less depression; increased their use of medical services, including diagnostic and preventive care known to improve health outcomes; and had less medical debt.[65] Given that 59 percent of uninsured African Americans live in states not extending Medicaid, compared to 44 percent of uninsured white people, there are clear racial inequities in terms of possibilities for improved access to care through Medicaid.[66]

Although the ACA was a significant policy shift, it represents a continuity with health care reforms made since the middle of the twentieth century. Briefly tracing reforms made since the Great Depression illustrates another set of disintegrating circuits that accrue capital through differentiating flows through valued and devalued bodies. These reforms have both expanded access to and consistently failed to include large segments of the population. Repeatedly, such reforms have entailed concessions to powerful elements of the private health care sector and powerful political blocs. Despite significant government spending, these concessions have entrenched power of the putatively private sector, arguably making fundamental reforms more difficult.

We can see this pattern established in the 1930s. President Roosevelt's Medical Advisory Committee identified national health insurance as an important part of creating economic security. Despite support from the American College of Surgeons, the American Medical Association (AMA) came out strongly against it.[67] In his 1935 message to Congress on Social Security, Roosevelt recommended increased federal aid to public health agencies but not health insurance, noting that "groups representing the medical profession are cooperating with the Federal Government in the further study of the subject and definite progress is being made."[68]

In conditions of major labor and social unrest during World War II, Roosevelt made health insurance an element of the Second Bill of Rights, which he proposed extending after the war.[69] With congressional limits on wage increases, unions were able to negotiate for health care as part of their collective bargaining agreements.[70] According to labor historian Alan Derickson, even as trade unions held a vision of universal, comprehensive health care, their negotiations for employer-based health insurance undermined future efforts to push for government interventions.[71] The expansion of private insurance through union contracts and employer benefit packages during and after the war largely benefited white workers.[72]

After World War II, Harry Truman pushed for the extension of comprehensive health insurance through the Social Security Administration, a reform that was successfully opposed using charges of socialized medicine. The Hill-Burton Act was passed in 1946 to fund hospital construction, and between 1947 and 1971, it provided $3.7 billion (along with $9.1 billion private funds) to private hospitals, which "virtually rebuilt America's private hospital system."[73] However, David Barton Smith observes, this was also the only piece of federal legislation passed in the twentieth century "that explicitly permitted the use of federal funds to provide racially exclusionary services."[74] Thus, it "institutionalized segregation where it had not existed and often accentuated the plight of the racially excluded African American patients and doctors throughout the South."[75]

By the late 1950s, growing medical costs created financial pressures on the elderly. This crisis converged with hospitals not being paid for their services to create a favorable context for reform. The passage of the Kerr–Mills Eldercare plan "marked the first time a compulsory health insurance bill of any kind" had been passed, but it did not take health care off the agenda during the 1960 presidential election.[76] Candidates Richard Nixon and John F. Kennedy both spoke of the need for health care reform, but it would not be until Lyndon Johnson's election after Kennedy's assassination that Medicare and Medicaid were passed. Many members of the AMA promised to boycott the program, but the legislation incorporated opponents through offering a flush revenue stream, which routed payments through existing insurance providers and reimbursed hospitals for their costs, including depreciation on new capital investments. This concession would fuel massive cost inflation in the sector, and it perversely undermined the financial viability of public hospitals across the country.[77]

In 1963, Black labor leader A. Philip Randolph told people gathered for the March on Washington: "Look for the enemies of Medicare, of higher minimum wages, of social security, of federal aid to education and there you will find the enemy of the Negro—the coalition of Dixiecrats and reactionary Republicans that seeks to dominate Congress."[78] The differences between Medicare and Medicaid illustrate some of Randolph's fears. While Medicare for all people over the age of sixty-five was a universal entitlement, states had tremendous latitude in the benefits they would offer and how many people would be covered under Medicaid. Medicaid thus represented a concession to Southern states that had failed to extend even minimal health and social services to poor and Black residents.

In the 1980s, President Ronald Reagan enacted a similar austerity agenda on welfare, antipoverty programs, and Medicaid that he had implemented as governor of California. The 1981 Omnibus Budget Reconciliation Act cut 25 percent from the budgets of most federal categorical health programs (such as neighborhood health centers) and implemented a rolling reduction of federal matching dollars to state Medicaid spending.[79] These cuts were followed in 1982 by a 10 percent reduction in Aid to Families with Dependent Children, resulting in 700,000 children being cut from Medicaid, and states made further Medicaid cuts during the recession.[80] Reforms implemented in the 1986 and 1987 Omnibus Budget Reconciliation Acts began a trend that would continue in coming years of delinking Medicaid from welfare, thereby opening the opportunity for states to enroll select categories of people (infants, pregnant women, people with disabilities, the elderly) with incomes between 100 percent and 185 percent of the poverty level.[81]

Reforms enacted between 1992 and 2010 evidence a crosscutting set of trends. President Clinton's proposal for health reform failed spectacularly, but he was able to pass the Children's Health Insurance Plan (CHIP) in 1997. This program was based on Medicaid, with joint state–federal funds to cover children whose families earned too much to qualify for Medicaid. Fifty percent more children were enrolled in Medicaid and CHIP over this time, and some states experimented with using waivers to extend eligibility to adults.[82] Between 1993 and 2010, health policy scholar Frank Thompson notes that there was also "considerable erosion in Medicaid's status as a formal legal entitlement" even as expenditures and the ratio of people enrolled to all poor people grew.[83]

These trends in part reflect what Thompson calls Medicaid's "entitlement paradox." Despite Medicaid's association with poverty and welfare, reforms enacted during this time worked to expand coverage, albeit unevenly, around categories of social deservingness, namely working families, middle-class families with family members who were elderly, and people living with disabilities.[84] The George W. Bush administration sought to rein in the CHIP program. Thompson writes:

> The White House sensed that a significant CHIP expansion that extended eligibility up the income ladder would fuel the program's progress in building a politically potent, middle-class constituency; it would thereby whet the public's appetite for government health insurance. Hence the White House worked to transform the debate over CHIP from a pragmatic give-and-take over how best to insure more children into a test of whether the country was on the road to "government-run health care" for all that would feature "a single-payer health system with rationing and price controls."[85]

This ideological effort would continue to animate conservative politics, but the line of social deservingness had been drawn farther up the income ladder in ways that insulated the program from attack.[86] By 2010, care for the elderly and disabled constituted two thirds of Medicaid spending, with over 70 percent of residents in nursing homes receiving Medicaid.[87]

Many poor and working-class people continued to be left out of Medicaid even as employer-based health insurance became far less common and more polarized. Between 1977 and 1996, the percentage of employer-based coverage for white workers fell from 77 percent to 71 percent while coverage for Black workers declined from 59 percent to 48 percent.[88] From 1980 to the early 2010s, people in the top two fifths of the income distribution faced an erosion of their benefits, but 90 percent retained their employer-based health coverage.[89] Over this same period, the percentage of people in the middle fifth income bracket not covered by workplace insurance increased from 5 percent to 12.4 percent. People whose incomes were lowest faced the sharpest losses of workplace coverage. While 10 percent of workers in the lower-middle fifth bracket were uninsured in 1980, this figure doubled to 21.9 percent in 2010; and for the poorest residents, the rate increased from 18 percent to 27.4 percent.[90]

With over 40 million people uninsured, and popular discontent over the recession and medical debt, President Obama sought to enact a comprehensive health reform. In 2007, health care costs had become a leading cause of bankruptcy, with 62 percent of personal bankruptcies resulting from medical debt.[91] Perhaps more importantly, health care costs continued to squeeze U.S. economic competitiveness: health care costs in 2010 comprised 17.7 percent of GDP compared to 11.5 percent for Germany, 10.1 percent for Japan, 9.6 percent for the United Kingdom, and 5.0 percent for China.[92] Obama's chief of staff, Rahm Emanuel, preferred an incremental approach, given his experience working under Clinton when his attempt at health care reform failed, but Obama regarded change as necessary for improving American economic competitiveness.[93]

Reform to a $2.6 trillion sector (nearly 17 percent of GDP) once again would require concessions.[94] David Axelrod, a senior advisor to Obama, remarked that accommodations were necessary to "get things done within the system as it is."[95] That is, the reform would not fundamentally alter the existing landscape of public sector funds flowing into private sector practice and profit, and thereby the disintegrating circuit. The American Hospital Association agreed to accept $155 million less in Medicare payments over ten years in exchange for an additional $171 billion in ACA-generated revenues, and the AMA similarly accepted payment reductions of $80 billion in exchange for $228 billion that the ACA's health expansion would generate.[96]

The geographic unevenness of Medicaid was well known. Indeed, as described above, geographic inequalities across and within states have deepened since the mid-1990s as states were given more latitude to enact waivers.[97] Authors of the ACA sought to build on this system with a proposal that might have led to greater equity across the states, and hence greater class and racial equity. As passed into law, the ACA increased the eligibility for Medicaid to everyone whose incomes fall below 133 percent of the federal poverty line and to those who do not have private insurance. Because Medicaid is run by the states, the federal government could not mandate extension, but the act did include enticements to participate, offering to pay 100 percent of the Medicaid expansion cost from 2014 to 2016, declining to 90 percent in 2020.[98]

Bill McCollum, Republican attorney general for the state of Florida, along with over twenty other states and the National Federation of Independent Businesses, sued the federal government over this provision.[99] Justice John Roberts's opinion in the 2012 Supreme Court opinion concluded that the federal government's inducement was "much more than 'relatively mild encouragement'—it is a gun to the head" because states stood to lose all of their existing Medicaid funding if they did not comply.[100] Roberts's use of the "gun to the head" analogy to characterize appropriations as coercion transferred emotional power to state actors who were not committed to ending the medical abandonment of their residents and the burden of debt, suicide, and poorer health they held. Indeed, the Roberts court ruling shored up both long-standing Southern states' rights prerogatives and neoconservative political geographies solidified in the Midwest and disproportionately white congressional districts.[101]

Still, opposition to Obamacare cannot be attributed only to conservative consolidation of whiteness through gerrymandered districts or lingering effects of Southern states' rights. Rather, the ACA and its opposition must be understood together within the history of bipartisan efforts to restructure welfare and health care by leveraging social unworthiness to consolidate social deservingness. The struggle over the ACA did not depart from decades of reforms that have simultaneously extended health care coverage and access and reproduced class and racial hierarchies. Those excluded from reform have been left to embody bad debt for which society refuses its obligations.

Conclusion: Empire's Displaced Violence

The debate over the ACA is haunted by the premature deaths of the past that continue to accumulate in the present; this reading is a way of grappling with and rejecting color-blind rationalizations of ongoing structural violence within racial capitalism. Following Jodi Melamed, "white is not what it was under white supremacist modernity. Rather, a formally antiracist, liberal-capitalist modernity has advanced to the point that well-off is the new white. [. . .] Whiteness (in the privileged form of multicultural whiteness) is deployed by neoliberal structures for profit making and for enhancing and augmenting its modes of accumulation."[102] With the futurity of whiteness at the discursive center of the suicide caucus discourse, conservative commentators failed to recognize how whiteness was not being threatened but rather consolidated through the ACA.

This circuit of accumulation accruing whiteness to capital and the well-off is what is missed by Rush Limbaugh's claim that the ACA is a form of reparations for past wrongs. His assertion that ACA would especially benefit the historically dispossessed anchors racism in the past, rendering the present as racially neutral. Yet not only do premature deaths that result from structural racism, capitalism, and imperial war making continue to accumulate in the present, but also the notion that the ACA could be considered a form of reparations violently distorts the meaning of the term. Even if one could ignore the additional public funds that will accumulate as private profit and not benefit all residents, groups who historically have been politically and economically dispossessed also explicitly have been targeted for exclusion. Indeed, Mark Meadows and his fellow Tea Party signatories grounded their opposition on the "state budget strains caused by Medicaid expansions."[103] Their efforts to "restore patient-centered healthcare in America" would hinge on excluding some people from the possibility of being patients.[104]

The broader Republican concern about political suicide was not about reckoning with or remedying the past but rather about retaining a tenuous hold on white supremacy within a shifting political geography of global capitalism. The Tea Party's discursive efforts to tether the ACA to sovereign debt, and hence the future of the nation, built on long-standing ideological efforts to attribute the federal deficit to a bloated government and excessive social spending, particularly on its entitlement programs. They leveraged the unspoken but racialized specter of the welfare queen to inveigh against the state. This tactic leverages race to obscure the fact that Medicare and Medicaid benefit socially deserving subjects, such as the elderly and children with special needs, and displaces discussion of corporate tax cuts and war as causes of sovereign debt.

Indeed, the debate over the ACA, debt, and reparations transpired in militarist terms while simultaneously displacing the harms of imperial war making. The *Atlantic* referred to the shutdown tactic as a "scorched-earth Republican offensive," and Obama accused the bloc of holding the American economy hostage, threatening to "burn down the house" and "blow up the entire economy."[105] California congressman Devin Nunes also drew explicit reference to war. By referring to the Tea Party bloc as "lemmings with suicide vests," Nunes spun the fiscal cliff metaphor to amplify Krauthammer's position that the shutdown tactic represented a losing battle.[106] The imagery of lemmings cast this group as unthinking and dangerous flock creatures whose blind ideological actions threatened to harm innocent parties.

The exceptional danger that the suicide bomber symbolizes rests on a racialized geopolitical imagination centering on the Middle East (Beirut, Iraq, Afghanistan). "The popular image," Mike Davis observes, "is that the typical suicide bomber is a simple-minded religious fanatic punching his admission ticket to a voluptuous afterlife."[107] Such violence is doubly illegitimate, undermining the state's claim to violence and symbolizing an external threat to the nation within Orientalist discourses.

Perhaps aware he had tread into too volatile a territory, Nunes attempted to minimize this external threat through reference to the John Hughes film *16 Candles*: "You guys remember Long Duk Dong at the end? That's going to be us tomorrow, waking up on the grass, crashed automobile. That's us."[108] Claiming for Americans the position of the harmless, drunken Chinese exchange student in a wealthy Chicago neighborhood tips the hat to another layer of Orientalist anxiety. What started as juvenile prank may in fact enable the Chinese government to call in U.S. sovereign debt! In situating the threat to carefree American consumption on China, Nunes displaces who pays the direct and indirect costs of Bush-era tax cuts and military operations in Afghanistan and Iraq (and many other places).[109]

These violent terms of debate largely went unremarked, registering as mere symbolic flourishes in the crisis pitch of rhetoric. I took note of them because of the disjuncture I saw between rhetorical references to martial sacrifice, hostage taking, and battlefield cowardice and the actual deaths from suicide among military veterans, people with medical and housing debt, and young people. Whose lives and futures were being mourned or leveraged? How could social debt (mutual responsibilities) be used to displace histories and present realities of racism and imperial war making, turning the most vulnerable into the irresponsible source of national crisis?

I have used Berlant's concepts of slow death and disintegrating circuits to think through how circuits of capital have been expanded through systemic exclusion from reform. I coupled this dwelling on sustained, everyday crisis with Gilmore's critical conceptualization of the materiality of racism and Gordon's concept of haunting to think about how prematurely ended lives weigh on the present. Where Berlant's slow death recognizes agency as laterally dispersed, Gordon's idea of haunting signals an intergenerational force or transfer of agency. For Gordon, "haunting, unlike trauma, is distinctive for producing a something-to-be-done."[110]

Premature deaths accumulate materially, but perhaps in a nonfinancial way, representing human losses that are unpayable but that remain social debts. As bluesologist Gil Scott-Heron once asked, "Who will pay reparations on my soul?" While lives violently undone cannot be remade, the marking of their unjust, violent absence demands action conceived differently than monetary repayment. At the risk of stating the obvious, the ACA cannot bring back the dead; nor does it represent the reparations that Limbaugh fears.[111] The ACA is haunted by historic patterns of racial and class exclusion; it does not signify repair understood as collective responsibility for present and future.[112] The vociferous opposition to the ACA by the Tea Party and continued through the 2016 election are driven by more than an ideological stance against big government, much less a principled, social justice critique of how the ACA funnels more public money to the private sector and fails to afford access to care to all. While many white people also face barriers to medical care, whiteness has effectively been tied to refusing debts of repair and mutual obligation. Indeed, so-called antiestablishment Republicans gathered popular backing through representing their efforts to dismantle the public sector as necessary to save the nation.

The social debt of a race-based medical system might be repaid with the extension of universal health care together with efforts to end individual and institutional racism in medicine. These would represent visceral, if modest, efforts toward healing and toward preventing further suffering and premature death. More broadly, health and social justice—another Reconstruction—would require remedies to historical and ongoing policies of dispossession and abandonment that harm so many rural and urban communities.[113] Broad-scale reinvestments in these places will require challenging how they are deployed ideologically as indebted threats to the economy, and hence the nation. Reparations might represent race-based medicine at the level of social healing—an effort to short-circuit the value that accrues from politically and economically disintegrating landscapes and institutions.

Coda

President-elect Donald J. Trump ran for office drawing on these same lines of racialized dispossession that brought Tea Party Republicans to political power a few years prior. He has not apologized for promoting the birther conspiracy theory and made dismantling Obamacare a central plank in his election campaign. The House Freedom Caucus, cofounded by Congress member Mark Meadows after the government shutdown, has continued its efforts to dismantle access to health care by targeting Planned Parenthood funding and has sent Trump a bucket list of 232 government regulations it would like the president to undo in his first 100 days in office, including rules regarding women's preventive health services; rules requiring Medicare and Medicaid providers to engage in emergency preparedness; regulations concerning confidentiality of patient records and protection of human subjects; eased work requirements for TANF recipients; and nondiscrimination protections for trans* and gender-nonconforming students.[114]

While there has been some debate on whether the Freedom Caucus will become irrelevant under a Trump administration, Trump has named one of its members, Rick Mulvaney, to head the Office of Management and Budget, and his other picks further suggest a sweeping commitment to dismantling government regulations and social protections. House Speaker Paul Ryan, while having clashed with candidate Trump and the Freedom Caucus, seems well positioned to push for turning Medicare into a voucher system and for supporting significant reforms to the ACA. Though far from universal health care, a repeal would double the number of uninsured people from 29 million in 2016 to 59 million—higher than before the ACA was implemented.[115]

If there is any bright spot on the congressional horizon, it is that a federal court ruled that the redistricting the GOP implemented in Wisconsin after the 2010 Tea Party sweep into government is unconstitutional—the first such ruling in decades.[116] Gerrymandering has arguably accelerated political polarization and the bodily disintegrating processes Berlant describes. This is evident, perhaps ironically, in polls of voters who say they oppose Obamacare yet support specific elements of the legislation. Race-based medicine as a system will be more firmly entrenched and reparations farther from political grasp.

Notes

1. Barrett Brown, "The Trouble with Charles Krauthammer," *Vanity Fair*, August 14, 2009. Charles Krauthammer, "Adventures in Identity Politics," *Real Clear Politics*, March 14, 2008, http://www.realclearpolitics.com/.

2. Krauthammer, "Adventures in Identity Politics."

3. I capitalize the category Black to signal how the term has been claimed as

part of a political project of self-determination. This usage also disturbs the idea that race somehow originates in skin color rather than how white supremacist ideologies have have used skin color to naturalize racism.

4. Dorothy Roberts, "Is Race-Based Medicine Good for Us? African-American Approaches to Race, Biomedicine, and Equality," *Journal of Law, Medicine, and Ethics* 36, no. 3 (2008): 539.

5. Emily Miller, "Boehner: ObamaCare Will Bankrupt Our Nation," *Human Events*, January 7, 2011, http://humanevents.com/.

6. Lawrence R. Jacobs and Theda Skocpol, *Health Care Reform and American Politics: What Everyone Needs to Know*, rev. ed. (New York: Oxford University Press, 2012), 15.

7. Mark Meadows, "Final House Defund Obamacare Letter," *Madison Project*, August 26, 2013, http://madisonproject.com/.

8. Sasha Abramsky, "How the Shutdown Hurts the Poor," *New Yorker*, October 8, 2013, http://www.newyorker.com/.

9. According to the Center on Budget and Policy Priorities, for the fiscal year 2015, safety net programs comprised 10 percent of federal spending; health insurance programs (Medicare, Medicaid, CHIP, and ACA subsidies) 25 percent; Social Security 24 percent; and defense 16 percent. The National Priorities Project breaks down these numbers slightly differently, distinguishing among mandatory spending (65 percent, with 23 percent for Medicare; 33 percent for Social Security; and the remainder for food assistance, unemployment, and all other); discretionary spending (29 percent, with 53.8 percent for military, 6 percent for education, 5.67 percent for housing and community, and remainder on all other), and debt (6 percent). "Policy Basics: Where Do Our Federal Tax Dollars Go?" *Center on Budget and Policy Priorities*, 2015, updated March 4, 2016, http://www.cbpp.org; "Federal Spending: Where Does the Money Go—Federal Budget 101," *National Priorities Project*, 2015, https://www.nationalpriorities.org.

10. Norman Daniels, Bruce Kennedy, and Ichiro Kawachi, *Is Inequality Bad for Our Health?* (Boston: Beacon Press, 2000); Richard G. Wilkinson, *Unhealthy Societies: The Afflictions of Inequality* (New York: Routledge, 2002); World Health Organization, *Closing the Gap in a Generation: Health Equity through Action on the Social Determinants of Health* (Geneva: World Health Organization, 2008); Ernest Drucker, *A Plague of Prisons: The Epidemiology of Mass Incarceration in America* (New York: New Press, 2013); Jenna M. Loyd, *Health Rights Are Civil Rights: Peace and Justice Activism in Los Angeles, 1963–1978* (Minneapolis: University of Minnesota Press, 2014); Michael Marmot and Jessica J. Allen, "Social Determinants of Health Equity," *American Journal of Public Health* 104 (suppl. 4) (2014): 517–19.

11. Jeanne Sahadi, "What's in the Fiscal Cliff?," *CNN Money*, November 9, 2012, http://money.cnn.com/.

12. David Edwards, "Fox News' Krauthammer: Cruz Leading Republican 'Suicide Caucus' by Opposing Obamacare," *Raw Story,* September 16, 2013, http://www.rawstory.com/.
13. Ibid.
14. David Edwards, "Ted Cruz: 'Why Is President Obama Threatening to Shut Down the Federal Government?,'" *Raw Story,* July 30, 2013, http://www.rawstory.com/; Byron York, "Ted Cruz Denies Saying 'Surrender Caucus'—The Record Says Otherwise," *Washington Examiner,* July 31, 2013, http://washingtonexaminer.com/.
15. "U.S. Shutdown Prompts Global Trepidation, Amusement," *GMA News,* October 3, 2013, http://www.gmanetwork.com/.
16. James Hookway, "Obama Shortens Asia Trip Due to Government Shutdown," *Wall Street Journal,* October 2 2013, http://online.wsj.com/.
17. Ryan Lizza, "Where the GOP's Suicide Caucus Lives," *New Yorker,* September 26, 2013, http://www.newyorker.com/.
18. Ibid.
19. Sabrina Tavernisena and Robert Gebeloff, "Millions of Poor Are Left Uncovered by Health Law," *New York Times,* October 2, 2013, http://www.nytimes.com/.
20. Ibid.
21. Lizza, "Where the GOP's Suicide Caucus Lives."
22. Ronald Brownstein, "Where Are the Uninsured Americans Who Will Benefit from Obamacare?," *Atlantic,* October 4, 2013, http://www.theatlantic.com/.
23. Jacobs and Skocpol, *Health Care Reform and American Politics,* 89–90.
24. Cedric J. Robinson, *Black Marxism: The Making of the Black Radical Tradition* (Chapel Hill: University of North Carolina Press, 1983); David T. Goldberg, *The Racial State* (Oxford: Blackwell Publishing, 2002).
25. David Harvey, *A Brief History of Neoliberalism* (Oxford: Oxford University Press, 2005).
26. David T. Goldberg, *The Threat of Race: Reflections on Racial Neoliberalism* (Malden, Mass.: Wiley-Blackwell, 2009), 363.
27. Ibid., 360, emphasis in original.
28. Paul Waldman, "Yes, Opposition to Obamacare Is Tied Up with Race," *Washington Post,* May 24, 2014, http://www.washingtonpost.com/.
29. Ibid.
30. Ibid.
31. Harriet Washington, *Medical Apartheid: The Dark History of Medical Experimentation on Black Americans from Colonial Times to the Present* (New York: Doubleday Books, 2006).
32. W. Michael Byrd and Linda A. Clayton, "The 'Slave Health Deficit': Racism and Health Outcomes," *Health/PAC Bulletin,* Summer 1991, 25–28; W. Michael

Byrd and Linda A. Clayton, *An American Health Dilemma: A Medical History of African Americans and the Problem of Race* (New York: Routledge, 2000); Rodney G. Hood, "The 'Slave Health Deficit': The Case for Reparations to Bring Health Parity to African Americans," *Journal of the National Medical Association* 93 no. 1 (2001): 1–5; Jewel Crawford, Wade W. Nobles, and Joy DeGruy Leary, "Reparations and Health Care for African Americans: Repairing the Damage from the Legacy of Slavery," in *Should America Pay? Slavery and the Raging Debate on Reparations*, ed. Raymond A. Winbush (New York: Harper Collins, 2003): 251–81.

33. Randall Robinson, *The Debt: What America Owes to Blacks* (New York: Plume, 2000); Iris Marion Young, *Responsibility for Justice* (Oxford: Oxford University Press, 2011); Alondra Nelson, *The Social Life of DNA: Race, Reparations, and Reconciliation after the Genome* (Boston: Beacon Press, 2016).

34. Lauren Berlant, *Cruel Optimism* (Durham, N.C.: Duke University Press, 2011), 105.

35. Ibid., 101.

36. Ibid., 104.

37. Ibid., 114.

38. Loyd, *Health Rights Are Civil Rights*.

39. *National Federation of Independent Business v. Sebelius*, Supreme Court 567 U.S. (2012), 6.

40. Andrew P. Wilper, Steffie Woolhandler, Karen E. Lasser, Danny McCormick, David H. Bor, and David U. Himmelstein, "Health Insurance and Mortality in U.S. Adults," *American Journal of Public Health* 99, no. 12 (2009): 2289–95.

41. Anne Case and Angus Deaton, "Rising Morbidity and Mortality in Midlife among White Non-Hispanic Americans in the 21st Century," *Proceedings of the National Academy of Sciences of the United States of America* 112, no. 49 (2015): 15078–83.

42. The figure of 400 "justifiable homicides" by police agents annually between 2008 and 2012 is from the FBI. The *Guardian* counted 500 deaths at hands of police in the first six months of 2015. No single federal agency counts deaths by police; Harvard social epidemiologist Nancy Krieger has called for public health agencies to report uniformly on these data. Alessandro De Giorgi, "Ferguson and Beyond: 'Justifiable Homicides' and Premature Death in the Urban Ghetto," *Social Justice*, August 21, 2014, http://www.socialjusticejournal.org/; Nancy Krieger, Jarvis T. Chen, Pamela D. Waterman, Mathew V. Kiang, and Justin Feldman, "Police Killings and Police Deaths Are Public Health Data and Can Be Counted," *PLOS Medicine* 12 (2015): e1001915, http://dx.doi.org/10.1371/journal.pmed.1001915.

43. Avery F. Gordon, *Ghostly Matters: Haunting and the Sociological Imagination*, 2nd ed. (Minneapolis: University of Minnesota Press, 2008), 17.

44. Ibid., 8.

45. Ruth Wilson Gilmore, *Golden Gulag: Prisons, Surplus, Crisis, and Opposition in Globalizing California* (Berkeley: University of California Press, 2006), 28.

46. W. E. B. Du Bois, *The Health and Physique of the Negro American* (Atlanta, Ga.: Atlanta University Press, 1906), 90.

47. Ibid.

48. M. Alfred Haynes, "The Gap in Health Status between Black and White Americans," in *Textbook of Black-Related Diseases*, ed. Richard A. Williams (New York: McGraw Hill, 1975), 8.

49. T. E. Malone and K. W. Johnson, *Report of the Secretary's Task Force on Black and Minority Health* (Washington, D.C.: U.S. Department of Health and Human Services, 1985). Thanks to Lorraine Halinka Malcoe for drawing my attention to this report, and for our conversations on health inequities related to health care.

50. Hood, "Slave Health Deficit."

51. Byrd and Clayton, "Slave Health Deficit," 28.

52. Arline T. Geronimus, John Bound, and Cynthia G. Colen, "Excess Black Mortality in the United States and in Selected Black and White High-Poverty Areas, 1980–2000," *American Journal of Public Health* 101, no. 4 (2011): 727.

53. Joseph G. Mangano, "Young Adults in the 1980s: Why Mortality Rates Are Rising," *Health/PAC Bulletin*, Summer 1991, 20.

54. Ibid., 22.

55. Ibid.

56. Geronimus, Bound, and Colen, "Excess Black Mortality," 720.

57. Ibid., 727.

58. Ibid.

59. Ibid., 728.

60. Commission to Build a Healthier America, "Beyond Health Care: New Directions to a Healthier America: Executive Summary," *Robert Wood Johnson Foundation*, 2009, http://www.commissiononhealth.org/PDF/11f12754-e8ff-408b-9451-6456d939b15f/ExecutiveSummary_FINAL.pdf, 7.

61. Dorothy Roberts, *Fatal Invention: How Science, Politics, and Big Business Re-create Race in the Twenty-First Century* (New York: New Press, 2011), 96–97.

62. Brian D. Smedley, Adrienne Y. Stith, and Alan R. Nelson, eds., *Unequal Treatment: Confronting Racial and Ethnic Disparities in Health Care* (Washington, D.C.: National Academies Press, 2003), 5.

63. Geiger's literature review covers studies conducted in the following categories of diagnosis and treatment: general medical and surgical care, coronary artery and other cardiac disease, cancer, cerebrovascular disease, asthma, renal disease and kidney transplantation, diabetes, HIV/AIDS, mental health, maternal and child health, and ophthalmic disease. H. Jack Geiger, "Racial and Ethnic Disparities

in Diagnosis and Treatment: A Review of the Evidence and Consideration of Causes," in *Unequal Treatment: Confronting Racial and Ethnic Disparities in Health Care,* ed. Brian D. Smedley, Adrienne Y. Stith, and Alan R. Nelson (Washington, D.C.: National Academies Press, 2003), 439–40.

64. Ibid., 442.

65. Sam Dickman, Danny McCormick, and Steffe Himmelstein, "Opting Out of Medicaid Expansion: The Health and Financial Impacts," *Health Affairs Blog,* January 30, 2014, http://healthaffairs.org/.

66. Kaiser Commission on the Uninsured, "Analyzing the Impact of State Medicaid Expansion Decisions," *Kaiser Family Foundation,* 2013, http://kaiserfamilyfoundation .files.wordpress.com/2013/07/8458-analyzing-the-impact-of-state-medicaid -expansion-decisions2.pdf.

67. Ezekiel J. Emanuel, *Reinventing American Health Care: How the Affordable Care Act Will Improve Our Terribly Complex, Blatantly Unjust, Outrageously Expensive, Grossly Inefficient, Error Prone System* (New York: Public Affairs, 2014), 131.

68. Franklin D. Roosevelt, "Message to Congress on Social Security," *Social Security Administration,* 1935, http://www.ssa.gov/history/fdrstmts.html#advisec.

69. Ira Katznelson, *Fear Itself: The New Deal and the Origins of Our Time* (New York: Norton, 2013), 196.

70. Laura A. Scofea, "The Development and Growth of Employer-Provided Health Insurance," *Monthly Labor Review,* March 1994, 6.

71. Alan Derickson, "Health Security for All? Social Unionism and Universal Health Insurance, 1935–1958," *Journal of American History* 80, no. 4 (1994): 1333–56.

72. Byrd and Clayton, *American Health Dilemma,* 149; George Lipsitz, *The Possessive Investment in Whiteness: How White People Benefit from Identity Politics* (Philadelphia: Temple University Press, 2005), 5.

73. Byrd and Clayton, *American Health Dilemma,* 205.

74. David Barton Smith, *Health Care Divided: Race and Healing a Nation* (Ann Arbor: University of Michigan Press, 1999), 47.

75. Byrd and Clayton, *American Health Dilemma,* 205.

76. Emanuel, *Reinventing American Health Care,* 138.

77. Loyd, *Health Rights Are Civil Rights,* 196–201.

78. Dona C. Hamilton and Charles V. Hamilton, *The Dual Agenda: Race and Social Welfare Policies of Civil Rights Organizations* (New York: Columbia University Press, 1997), 127.

79. Geraldine Dallek, "Frozen in Ice: Federal Health Policy during the Reagan Years," *Health/PAC Bulletin,* Summer 1988, 4.

80. Ibid.

81. Ibid., 5.

82. Frank J. Thompson, *Medicaid Politics: Federalism, Policy Durability, and Health Reform* (Washington, D.C.: Georgetown University Press, 2012), Loc. 1988.
83. Ibid., Loc. 4474.
84. Ibid., Loc 4628.
85. Ibid., Loc. 1880.
86. Alaska governor Sarah Palin and other conservatives did try to link health reforms to rationing and government-sponsored "death panels" in the 2008 elections. Emanuel, *Reinventing American Health Care*, 168–69.
87. Thompson, *Medicaid Politics*, Loc. 2223, 2249.
88. Jon R. Gabel, "Job-Based Health Insurance, 1977–1998: The Accidental System under Scrutiny," *Health Affairs* 18 no. 6 (1999): 65.
89. Jacobs and Skocpol, *Health Care Reform and American Politics*, 19.
90. Ibid.
91. Ibid., 27, 200.
92. "Health Expenditure, Total (% GDP)," *World Bank*, 2014, http://data.worldbank.org/indicator/SH.XPD.TOTL.ZS.
93. Jacobs and Skocpol, *Health Care Reform and American Politics*, 44.
94. Marilyn W. Serafini, "National Health Spending Grew Slowly in 2010," *Kaiser Health News*, January 9, 2012, http://www.kaiserhealthnews.org/.
95. Jacobs and Skocpol, *Health Care Reform and American Politics*, 68.
96. Ibid., 70.
97. Thompson, *Medicaid Politics*, Loc. 2594, 4494.
98. Emanuel, *Reinventing American Health Care*, 208–9.
99. Jacobs and Skocpol, *Health Care Reform and American Politics*, 152; Emanuel, *Reinventing American Health Care*, 189.
100. *National Federation of Independent Business v. Sebelius*, 51.
101. Lizza, "Where the GOP's Suicide Caucus Lives."
102. Jodi Melamad, *Represent and Destroy: Rationalizing Violence in the New Racial Capitalism* (Minneapolis: University of Minnesota Press, 2011), 223.
103. Meadows, "Final House Defund Obamacare Letter."
104. Ibid.
105. Brownstein, "Where Are the Uninsured Americans?"; Scott Neuman, "President to GOP: Don't 'Burn Down the House,'" *NPR*, September 27, 2013, http://www.npr.org/.
106. Rosalind S. Helderman, "Nunes Calls Fellow House Republicans 'Lemmings with Suicide Vests,'" *Washington Post*, September 30, 2013, http://www.washingtonpost.com/.
107. Mike Davis, *Buda's Wagon: A Brief History of the Car Bomb* (London: Verso, 2007), 98.
108. Helderman, "Nunes Calls."
109. Kathy Ruffling and Joel Friedman, "Economic Downturn and Legacy of

Bush Policies Continue to Drive Large Deficits," *Center on Budget and Policy Priorities*, February 28, 2013, http://www.cbpp.org/.

110. Gordon, *Ghostly Matters*, Loc. 201.

111. Ta-Nehisi Coates, "The Case for Reparations," *Atlantic*, June 2014, http://www.theatlantic.com/.

112. Young, *Responsibility for Justice*.

113. Loyd, *Health Rights Are Civil Rights*.

114. House Freedom Caucus, *First 100 Days: Rules, Regulations, and Executive Orders to Examine, Revoke, and Issue,* December 14, 2016, https://meadows.house.gov/.

115. Judith Solomon, "Republican Health Reform Repeal Plan Would Leave 30 Million More Uninsured," *Center on Budget and Policy Priorities,* December 7, 2016, http://www.cbpp.org.

116. Michael Wines, "Judge Finds Wisconsin Redistricting Unfairly Favored Republicans," *New York Times,* November 21, 2016, http://www.nytimes.com/.

4

Bidil's Compensation Relations

ANNE POLLOCK

When BiDil, the medication for heart failure in "self-identified black patients," was introduced to the market, it was met with great fanfare. Proponents celebrated the pill, indicating that as the first medication specifically for African Americans, it was taking important steps in remedying hundreds of years of inadequate care for that group. Opponents denounced it, emphasizing the dubious history of racial profiling in medicine and pointing out that such drugs would unjustly profiteer from African American patients.[1] A consensus held that BiDil would be a tremendous market success. Yet it wasn't: BiDil flopped.[2] Its impact in the broader pharmaceutical industry was insignificant, and other drugs geared to racialized populations have not followed.

This pill, although a small player in the market, provides an important opportunity for analysis of the complex dynamics of debt within the health care system and the related lack of attention to the broader, racially stratified society. These dynamics of debt need to be understood through the lens of the regimes of value. Monetary value is perhaps the most familiar such regime, but race and medicine are necessarily also intertwined with other modes of value, including epistemological, ethical, moral, and political.[3] At the same time, monetary value is more complex than a price tag. Many analysts have put BiDil into the context of market-driven medicine, which is an important first step for considering its relationship with debt.[4] However, the discussion can be simultaneously broadened and deepened by paying attention to how monetary value was ascribed to BiDil and yet in significant ways was unrealized. This analysis shows that the concern about the high cost of the pill held by opponents of BiDil is based on the same flawed thinking as that of proponents of

BiDil, who believed the pill would positively affect access to health care. Both failed to take into account the complex relationships between the various players, as well as how that fit into the social and political context within which the pill came to market, and failed.

Because BiDil has been a commercial failure, its debts are hard to track: they are not easily monetized or placed in a ledger. Nevertheless, debt is a heterogeneous and slippery concept that vacillates between the monetary and the moral, and it remains relevant. Relatedly, markets are not simple things but rather sites of relationships. As the dominant site of monetary exchange, markets are a key space of debt—where debts might be accrued, repaid, mediated, carried over, or discharged. Markets are also social spheres in which monetary value is mediated. Markets do not determine drugs' use value—which is to say their efficacy—but the inability to access drugs in the market prevents any use value from being realized. Not all recognized debts successfully compel repayment. The ability to extract compensation, for a debt or otherwise, depends on the broader socially situated relationships at play.

Here I use the marketing, and market failure, of the most prominent example of race-based medicine, BiDil, to show how the nonalignment of regimes of value matters for understanding racialized medicine in the United States today. I analyze the marketing of BiDil first, then put these marketing materials into the context of broader issues of compensation relations around BiDil, both before and after the drug's approval. Compensation relations is a concept that seeks to track not only debt ledgers but also the lines of value transfers—that is, relations between the pharmaceutical company and the physicians that performed the trial on the one hand, and the U.S. Food and Drug Administration (FDA) that approved its race-based indication on the other; and between the pharmaceutical company and patients as mediated through the complex array of public and private payers. Compensation relations are in part characterized by debt, but debt by itself does not guarantee the ability to extract payment. That depends on power and on positioning within networks.

Using the frame of compensation relations to examine race-based medicine shifts the focus from the debt caused by an expensive drug to an inability to extract compensation. This sheds light on the complex dynamics of power that exist between the many actors in the pharmaceutical industry as well as the impact of social factors, such as those experienced by underserved populations. Once again, this places the pill within its broader social and political context, and it emphasizes that BiDil is just one small aspect of this terrain and its racialization. In broadening the notion of debt to that of compensation relations, this analysis expands the sphere of actors from a unilateral relationship between a pharmaceutical company and Black patients to complex relationships between different players in the pharmaceutical industry: pharmaceutical companies, medical associations, government regulators, public and private insurers, and underserved Black patients.

We should resist the assumption, taken for granted in much critique of pharmaceutical companies and marketing, that marketing and compensation efforts are effective in getting the pharmaceutical company what it wants. Insofar as the debate about race-based medicine has addressed markets, it has generally operated on an idealized notion of markets, in which the entire target market purchases the drug at its advertised price. If we fail to take into account how limited the pharmaceutical company behind BiDil has been in guiding medical practice and determining patient experience, we fail to understand racialized medicine as it is in the world: how it moves through markets, and how it transforms bodies. The commercial failure of the first drug with a racial indication is as important a part of the terrain of racialized medicine as are its initial approval and marketing. At the same time, the racialization of medicine does not rise or fall on this particular pill; rather, it exists, and will continue to exist, in the context of complex, nuanced relationships between actors in the pharmaceutical industry and in broader society.

How BiDil Came to Market

When BiDil was approved by the FDA in 2005 with the controversial indication for heart failure in "self-identified black patients," it became the first drug with a racially specific indication. The clinical trial that led to BiDil's approval, the African-American Heart Failure Trial (A-HeFT), specifically enrolled only Black patients, and the pharmaceutical company sought a race-specific approval because that indication had a longer remaining patent life.[5] A-HeFT compared standard-of-care treatment plus placebo with standard-of-care treatment plus a new combination of two drugs already available as generics for other indications: isosorbide dinitrate was indicated for chest pain, hydralazine was indicated for hypertension, and A-HeFT tested a combination of the two for heart failure. In A-HeFT, BiDil's drug combination added to standard heart failure treatment was so convincingly beneficial for lowering the risk of death that the trial was ended early.[6] Because A-HeFT did not compare different racial groups, the trial did not actually prove race-specific efficacy. I will return to the FDA's decision to apply the unusual racially specific indication that the drug company sought, but at the outset it is also worth noting that the trial showed the efficacy of the drug combination in patients with access to it.

At the time of BiDil's approval, both its proponents and its vocal critics predicted impending profits.[7] However, the drug was a market failure, reaching only a single-digit percentage of its target population in the years after its release; the company that originally owned the patent on it, NitroMed, ceased marketing the drug and laid off most of its staff in 2008.[8] A new company has bought the patent and has been modestly restarting marketing since 2012, but as a market object, BiDil is a pale shadow of what it was widely anticipated to be.[9] Pharmaceuticalization literature generally highlights the expansive capacities of drugs, but failed drugs offer an opportunity to explore socially structured constraints.[10]

It seems fair to say that BiDil has been on some level a marketing failure, yet its marketing materials are still rich fodder for analysis. The original 2005 marketing plan for BiDil combined the usual outreach to relevant physicians with partnerships with the NAACP and the Congressional Black Caucus and community outreach through churches, barbershops, and Black newspapers.[11] This was an unusual approach, and one out of step with Big Pharma, which overwhelmingly focuses on marketing to physicians.[12] The physician focus is even true of major blockbuster drugs that also have expensive direct-to-consumer advertising on TV. BiDil was the product of a small pharma firm, and the community emphasis seems to have been part of an effort to market on the cheap. There has also been some suggestion that the relatively small budget for marketing was misspent. According to a business publication exploring what should be learned from BiDil's market failure (which draws on interviews with key individuals involved with the science and marketing), more money was spent on salaries than on actual marketing.[13] There is little left to show for the marketing budget outlay.

Rather than hire a marketing company that was well established in the pharmaceutical space, NitroMed hired Vigilante, a division of Publicis that describes itself as "a leading urban marketing firm that specializes in advertising targeted to young, multi-cultural audiences in the urban market" that combines "traditional advertising media" with "grass roots marketing and interactive media."[14] The firm is best known for splashy marketing for major corporations: Vigilante's then top executive was the one who "conceived of and implemented the Oprah Car Giveaway[,] heralded by some as being the biggest single day promotion in the history of advertising."[15] Experience in capturing the attention of young consumers is not necessarily useful for marketing a drug for heart failure. Moreover, it matters that selling pharmaceuticals is quite different from selling cars,

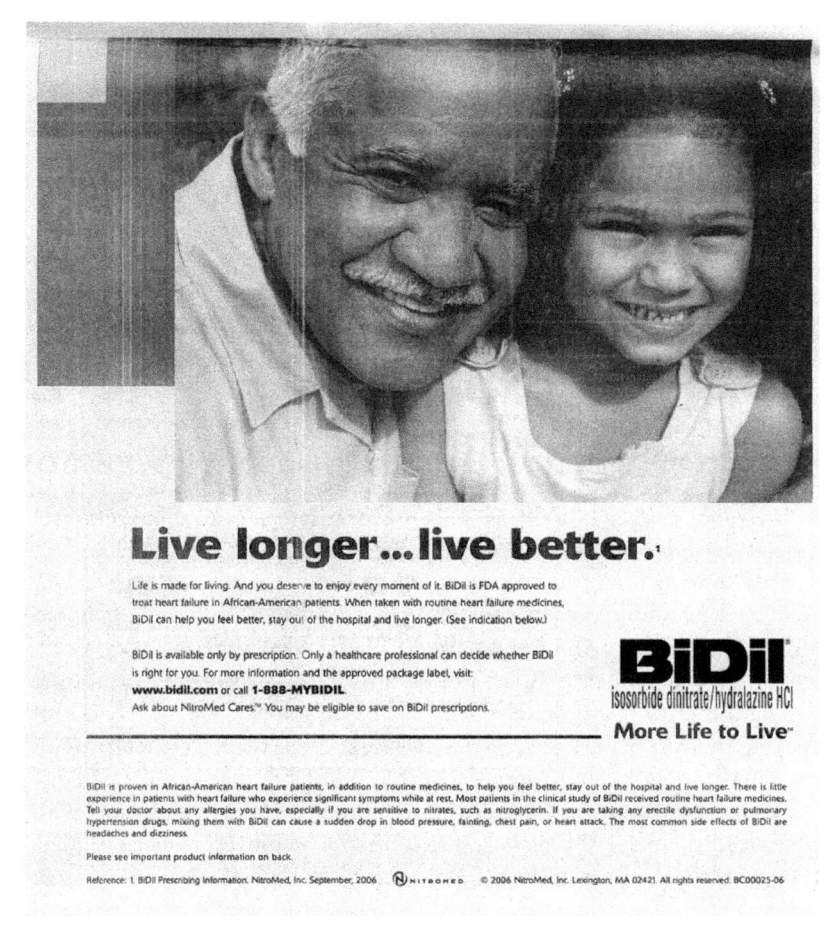

Figure 4.1. This advertisement, showing an older man of color and a young girl, was part of BiDil's direct-to-consumer marketing campaign. Printed in the *Washington Afro-American,* October 6–13, 2006, 6.

and their ads and broader public relations campaign for BiDil did not break through.

The print ads that appeared for BiDil (Figure 4.1) in African American newspapers in Washington, D.C., and other cities with large African American populations come across like knockoffs of conventional direct-to-consumer ads. Much of the space of the ad is taken up by an image of an older man of color who is smiling together with a little girl. The large text has the vague promise, "Live longer . . . live better," and the regular-sized text keeps things general: "Life is made for living. And you deserve to enjoy every moment of it." Both the racial indication and the disease indication are treated with a light touch: "BiDil is FDA approved to treat heart failure in African-American patients. When taken with routine heart failure medicines, BiDil can help you feel better, stay out of the hospital and live longer." The text continues with only slightly out of the ordinary wording, insofar as it recommends talking to your "health care professional" rather than "your doctor"—perhaps an acknowledgment that many patients, especially among underserved populations, are treated by nurse practitioners and other nonphysicians: "BiDil is available only by prescription. Only a healthcare professional can decide whether BiDil is right for you." The ad gives a Web address and phone number, and it notes that the company has a program to offer discounts: "Ask about NitroMed Cares™. You may be eligible to save on BiDil prescriptions." The small print includes a few caveats, including risks of mixing with erectile dysfunction drugs. This print campaign is so unambitiously conceived that it seems almost pro forma.

This limited direct-to-consumer advertising component was an adjunct to the community outreach and mass publicity focus that anchored BiDil's marketing.[16] All of these approaches underestimated how structurally underserved the BiDil population is—for example, the target population disproportionately lacks insurance or resources to pay out of pocket, and disproportionately receives care from overstretched providers who are less likely to implement the latest findings of cutting-edge research or to navigate complicated reimbursement schemes (and who are indeed skeptical about the value of race-based medicine[17]). The marketing approach operated on the assumption that African American heart failure patients and their communities could and would drive demand themselves, without regard for the mediation of the market through prescribers and payers—key aspects of compensation relations, which I will return to below.[18]

By 2013, the BiDil website constituted the modest Web presence of the drug (Figure 4.2). Like most pharmaceutical websites, it was divided into sections for health care providers and for patients. The side for providers was illustrated by an African American man in a white coat and draped with a stethoscope, and the side for patients was illustrated by an older African American couple smiling with a bicycle. As is conventional for pharmaceutical advertising, the image chosen to represent patients was of people who look healthy, not of people who look different because of their disease.[19] There is an absurdity in putting a trim woman on a bicycle

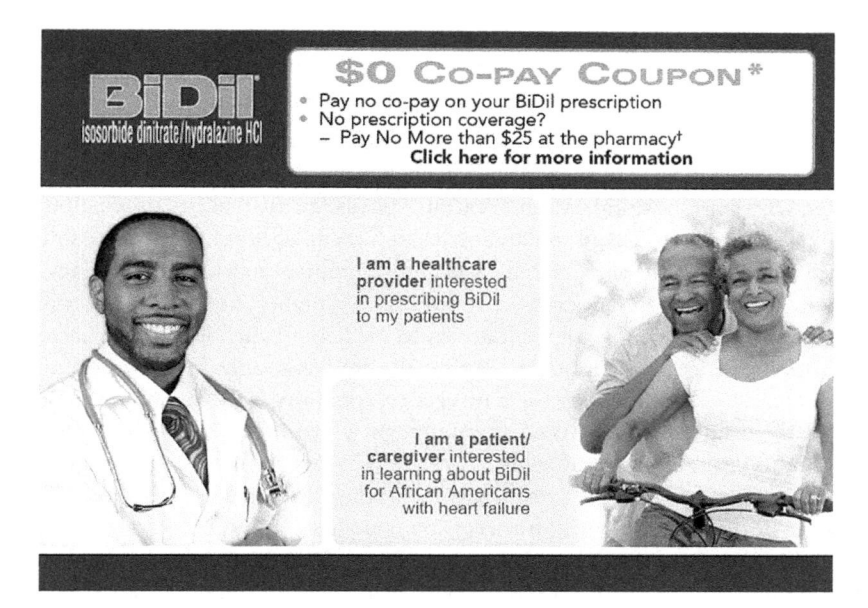

Figure 4.2. This screen capture of BiDil's website home page (BiDil.com) shows images of African Americans in the sections for health care providers and patients.

in an ad for heart failure, but it is one that is consistent with direct-to-consumer marketing generally. It is notable that the images of both the health care provider and the patients are apparently African American. The choice to represent the doctor as African American may be a cynical effort to undercut criticism that the drug is an extension of racist power relations in medicine, or it may be an implicit reference to the Association of Black Cardiologists (ABC), who played a key role in the study that led to BiDil's approval.

Yet I am even more interested in an aspect of the page that is less visually rich. An intriguing piece of promotional media appeared as a banner on top of the Web page, before and after clicking whether one is seeking information as a health care provider or as a patient or caregiver: $0 copay coupon for BiDil (Figure 4.3).[20] The coupon itself is quite different from a community outreach event or even the conventional direct-to-consumer imagery. The coupon has no images of people, but there are many relationships built in.

What does a $0 copay coupon mean? First of all, note that a $0 copay coupon is not the same as free drugs. As anthropologists of global health have pointed out, drug distribution has costs for patients and for providers even when the drugs themselves are free.[21] The cost of accessing the coupon for an individual patient is much more than the copay—and not only in the most immediate sense of requiring access to the Internet and particular kinds of literacy. Using the coupon requires a clinical encounter, whether a hospitalization event or a physician visit, either of which is likely to cost the patient much more than $25, in addition to the time and transport and other associated costs. It also requires a visit to a pharmacy, with its own attendant costs. The coupon highlights the fact that access to health insurance is not itself access to medicine, much less health care.

Another noteworthy detail is that the $0 fee is only for insured patients, which means that their insurance company is paying something for the drug. There is also an alternative provided for uninsured patients. Qualifying uninsured patients must pay $25 per month—a reasonably modest amount, but not zero. This is another way in which the coupon does not provide the drug for free; someone has to pay.

Even as the Affordable Care Act (ACA, or Obamacare) has expanded the number of African Americans with health insurance, it has not eliminated Black–White disparities in insurance coverage,[22] and any particular insurance policy may decide not to cover a drug. Resistance on the part of insurance companies foreshadowed a broader trend prominent in the wake of the ACA: pharmaceutical companies must not only shield their patients from the true cost of the drug, as they have historically done by passing the price on to insurers, but they must prove its value to payers.[23] This kind of coupon can be read as a tactic to shield the patient from the cost of the drug even if the insurer does not think that the drug is worth the price. With the ascendance of coupons for prescription drugs since the 2008 financial crisis, there has been increasing criticism of the costs that coupons for brand-name drugs add for insurers and to the health care system as a whole, and for patients once coupon programs end.[24] A coupon is issued at the discretion of the pharmaceutical company; it is thus intrinsically insecure as a mode of access. From the perspective of a pharmaceutical company, one motivation for providing a coupon is to instill brand loyalty: once patients begin taking BiDil, they are more likely to try to stay on it rather than to seek out generic equivalents or to do without. Thus, coupons (like free samples) are often short term by design. On a more macroeconomic level, pharmaceutical companies are motivated to offer "free" or discounted drugs for the purposes of protecting competitive advantage: if the drug is available to price-sensitive consumers at little or no cost, it is difficult for generic companies to gain

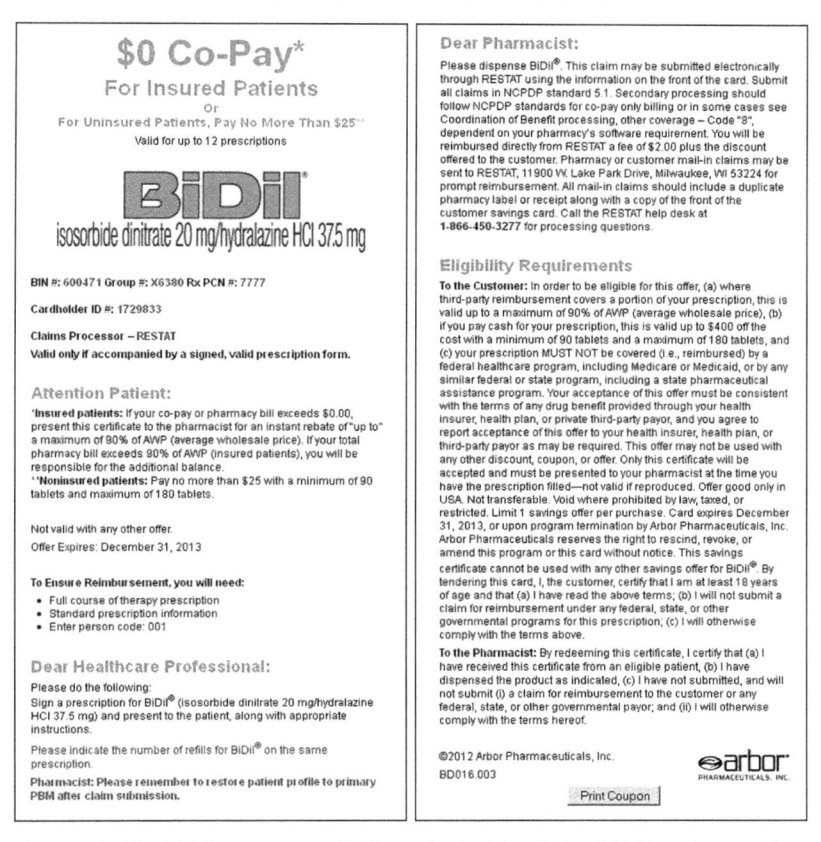

Figure 4.3. The BiDil coupon, available on the BiDil website (BiDil.com), offered a $0 copay.

market share. More abstractly, coupons like this provide moral cover for high prices. Giving limited access to "free" drugs can thus be part of pricing strategies to maintain high prices while providing cover in the face of moral criticism for profiteering from the suffering of the poor.[25]

This coupon draws our attention to the fact that the copay for BiDil can be relatively high because it has often not been given preferred status in formularies. Formularies are lists of drugs that particular insurance policies will pay for, and the popular model of tiered formularies encourages patients to select particular drugs from the list by charging the patient a lower copay for preferred drugs and a higher copay for drugs that are considered to be less cost-effective. In theory, high copayments for BiDil would encourage the use of generic equivalents. That generally works for newly generic drugs that effectively inherit the marketing of the brand-name drug that they are copying; this is part of how generic companies engage in a process of "unbranding."[26] However, that common situation was not present here because the old generic drugs combined in BiDil were to be prescribed for a new indication. This unusual market route created challenges for both the brand and the generic alternatives. Because BiDil's components were available as generics, there was a plausible rationale to put the brand on the formularies' nonpreferred list. Cobbled-together combinations of the generic chest pain drug isosorbide dinitrate and the hypertension drug hydralazine could not ride on the coattails of BiDil because they were not indicated for use in heart failure (in African Americans or otherwise). Thus, formularies' incentive structures more often led simply to nonadoption of the therapy rather than to generic substitution. Suffice it to say that the relatively high copay for BiDil became a barrier to its adoption—one that coupons like this one sought to overcome. This aspect of the drug's cost is where many might focus a discussion of debt and race-based medicine. However, this myopic focus on the cost of the drug misses the larger cost of race-based medicine to African American communities and to society as a whole.

Compared to the direct-to-consumer print ads and community outreach campaigns that inaugurated BiDil, this coupon represents the recent streamlining of discounts and negotiations with insurers. It can be read as a shift in the primary target of the extraction of value: from patients to payers. Health care providers who write prescriptions—physicians, physician assistants, and nurse practitioners—play a key mediating role in both marketing models, but one that shifts. Analysis of how patients, prescribers, and payers are configured in BiDil's marketing provides an opportunity to grapple with the political economy of racialized pharmaceuticals in the United States.

This coupon does not necessarily address debt per se. It does not play a decisive role in imposing or relieving monetary burden, and it does not absolve the moral burden of caring for patients in need. What it does highlight is the difficulty in extracting compensation not only from underserved patients but also from third-party payers. The conventional answer for why BiDil was a commercial failure was that it was priced too high, but it makes more sense to consider it a failure to extract compensation. This coupon is a modest attempt to operate on the compensation relation—an attempt that ultimately failed. BiDil's failure to extract compensation is directly linked to its commercial failure.

BiDil's Broader Compensation Relations

These relationships of compensation deserve fuller explanation. The etymology of compensation is "weighing against." Compensation tells us nothing about intrinsic value. Compensation more than debt highlights the fact that payback might be in a different regime of value, especially as it emerges in legal contexts—money for time, money for services, money for the endurance of harm. Debt is a way of describing what is owed; compensation is a way to characterize what is actually given.

There are layers of debt as well as compensation relations in BiDil. In the case of BiDil, who owes what to whom, and where did it break down? A few of the main players were NitroMed, its shareholders, the ABC, the state (which is actually plural—the FDA and state payers [Medicare and Veterans Affairs]), and Black patients with heart failure. Each of these categories of actors is in debt and compensation relationships with each other. The compensation relation between NitroMed and Black patients is not necessarily direct; it is a highly mediated relation and is not itself a primary locus of extraction of value. So who and what comes between NitroMed and Black patients with heart failure?

NitroMed was in a compensation relation with its shareholders. In dollar terms, the major extraction of value was from investors, who lost out as NitroMed's share price dropped from a peak of $20 a share to a buyout at 80 cents a share.[27] The BiDil patent is now owned by a private company, Arbor Pharmaceuticals, so we can't put a numeric value on it in the same way, but suffice it to say that the value is low. The shareholders have largely fallen out of the story of BiDil, which is of course not necessarily a bad thing if we are concerned with health as a public good.

NitroMed was also in a compensation relation with the ABC, whom the company paid $200,000 to help run the trial that led to BiDil's approval.[28] It also made donations to ABC and other organizations that do advocacy for African Americans. For example, it gave the NAACP a $1.5 million grant to support efforts to improve health care for African Americans.[29] Although some analysts have suggested that these financial transactions bought off these organizations, I would argue that it's fairer to say that the ABC and the NAACP, in a limited way and with an independent voice, bought in.[30] Moreover, we should not take for granted which direction the primary extraction of value goes: both the ABC and the NAACP survive in a much more robust form than does NitroMed, which has been liquidated.

The compensation relations of various parties with the federal government are complex. In the first place, the federal government is plural: the

FDA and the Congressional Black Caucus are on the upstream side, and payers such as Medicare and Veterans Affairs are closer to the patients. NitroMed made payments to the upstream federal players. It is standard FDA policy that pharmaceutical companies seeking approval pay fees to expedite review,[31] and the FDA lists NitroMed as a company that has made successful use of this policy.[32] NitroMed also gave money to the Congressional Black Caucus, whose members played important roles at the FDA hearing on BiDil. Noting this compensation should be the beginning of the analysis, not the end.

One question raised in this volume is about the moral debt of the government to its minority subjects, and this resonates with elements of the FDA hearing that led to BiDil's approval. Moral debt was invoked by the Congressional Black Caucus speaker at the FDA hearings on BiDil, Donna Christensen, the first public speaker invited to comment:

> I am here before you this afternoon as Chair of the Health Braintrust of the Congressional Caucus, and I want to say to you that today, ladies and gentlemen, you have before you an unprecedented opportunity to significantly reduce one of the major health disparities in the African American community and, in doing so, to begin a process that will bring some degree of equity and justice to the American health care system.[33]

Christensen went on to describe disparities in heart disease and the possible role of nitrous oxide. She spoke of the reason to support the racial indication as a way to acknowledge the courage of the pharmaceutical company in looking at the signal in the earlier trials and doing a new trial in Blacks, a risky decision that deserved to be rewarded:

> The position at the CBC on the approval of BiDil is clear and unequivocal. It should be approved and indicated for use in African Americans. We are only cognizant of the many social, political and economic variance which define being an African American in the United States today. Addressing these in eliminating the disparities that exist in all aspects of our lives is our highest priority until those gaps are closed. Their continued existence despite our best efforts must not be used to deny treatment to those for whom treatment has been denied and deferred for four hundred years. Today this panel is being asked to reverse that history.[34]

This public comment is important for understanding what was going on in the compensation relation between the pharmaceutical company and the FDA. Christensen's articulation is resonant with claims made in terms of what anthropologist Adriana Petryna has called biological citizenship: "a massive demand for but selective access to a form of social welfare based on medical, scientific, and legal criteria that both acknowledge biological injury and compensate for it."[35] Biological citizenship is a key lens through which Jonathan Xavier Inda has compellingly argued that BiDil was involved in "materializing hope."[36] Yet it matters that here the compensation is not given directly to patients but to the pharmaceutical company as their proxy. Moreover, the compensation from the FDA to NitroMed is not in cash but in a different regime of value.

The comments from the chair of the FDA panel, Steve Nissen, highlighted the indirectness of the compensation. He spoke in a way that resonated with Christensen's call to address long-standing health disparities, albeit in more clinical terms, and translated the obligation to the patients into obligation to the pharmaceutical company (here "the sponsor"):

> Do you get points for doing a study in people for which it is more difficult to do the study and where the information is very valuable from a societal point of view and from a medical care point of view? You know, I live in Cleveland, Ohio, Bob. We have a very large African American population. We see a lot of heart failure. As we all know and we are to talk about a little bit later, ACE [angiotensin-converting enzyme] inhibitors don't work so well in that population. So, when you get information that is potentially very valuable and informative about a group that can be very difficult to treat, you have to give a sponsor some points for going after that.[37]

Like Christensen, Nissen framed BiDil as compensating for past and ongoing neglect. He also framed BiDil as a way to address the (questionable) claim that African Americans do not respond to other treatments for heart failure, as compensation for a more narrowly pharmaceutical lack, and as a way to get African Americans to participate in clinical trials:

> You know, it is hard [to enroll African Americans in trials] for some of the reasons you heard from the microphone today. That is, there is distrust of the health provider community by African Americans, some of it justified. So, we have to overcompensate in order to make people comfortable in minority groups with participating in clinical trials. Now, we are working at that and we are doing a lot of work to try to do that. These folks were able to pull it off and I am going to give them some points for that.[38]

Nissen used the term "overcompensation" and spoke of giving points: compensating for lack of effective drugs and for lack of representation in trials. Interestingly, Nissen does not simply blame African American distrust on individually held ideas based on historical wrongs, as many invocations of distrust do, but rather suggests that health care providers need to do something differently in the present.[39] He recognizes the value of doing the work that it takes to build trust with African American trial participants. Yet the FDA's control over monetary compensation is ultimately limited. The FDA does not give money directly to pharmaceutical companies. In this case, Nissen's point giving did not accomplish another mode of compensation necessary for the pharmaceutical company to realize the value of its intellectual property: from payers—whether patients or their public or private insurers—to the pharmaceutical company.

According to Christensen and Nissen, the government had accrued debts in this case; it had obligations to minority communities, and it had accrued debt to the pharmaceutical company that took the time and trouble to find something useful for those patients. In the terms of their intervention, the FDA became the agency of the government that bore the obligation. Yet the FDA is only one actor among many setting the terms of compensation relations. Even "the government" is not just one thing.

Key members of and other speakers at the FDA panel articulated an obligation to approve BiDil as a race-based pharmaceutical to compensate NitroMed for its research, but many parts of "the government" did not come to bear the obligation to compensate BiDil's maker. For example, the key payers of Medicare and Veterans Affairs decided that generic substitution would be acceptable in this case, and they put BiDil in a tier of drugs with higher copays and thus less access. Because drug coverage for older people is covered through special Medicare Part D plans rather than through Medicare itself, and in the absence of guidance from the Center for Medicare and Medicaid Services (CMS) that BiDil should be covered by Medicare Part D plans, NitroMed had to negotiate with each plan for coverage, which was slow to come.[40] Many government payers did not feel that they owed this race-based medicine to African American patients. From the perspective of some advocates, this amounted to CMS "undermining the patent system."[41] Worth underscoring here is that the government is heterogeneous: the FDA effectively acknowledged that it owed, but Medicare and Veterans Affairs did not follow suit.

Nissen made a gesture toward owing Black patients, and he compensated the pharmaceutical company as a proxy. That this compensation failed to reach its target patients is beyond his purview. He can help the drug to reach the market, but from there, the drug's movement is beyond his control. As Jonathan Xavier Inda has pointed out with regard to the commercial failure of BiDil, "The market works only for those who have the ability to pay."[42] Inda compellingly argues that BiDil's commercial failure "speaks to the corporal abandonment under neoliberalism of people who lack the financial wherewithal to purchase medical and other goods necessary to achieve proper health."[43] Both state actors and private actors are implicated in this abandonment.

This failure of BiDil to command compensation in the market helps us to see that one of the widespread worries about BiDil during the lead-up to its approval and in the immediate wake of its release was a misapprehension: the idea was that, by rebranding generic components as a high-price branded pill, BiDil would raise the cost of drugs for Black patients. This concern has been highlighted by many academic analysts. For example, in one typical framing, Duana Fullwiley describes the problem of BiDil as "race-tailored therapy [that] has dramatically increased cost for the racial group it claims to benefit."[44] Yet experience contradicts this characterization: because patients are overwhelmingly not receiving BiDil, they are obviously not paying its cost. Moreover, the idea that BiDil would necessarily increase the prescription costs for African Americans is also an oversimplification of the economics at stake. At the most basic level, the list price of any given prescription drug is not the same as the cost that patients themselves pay for it. If insurers, including Medicare, had been willing to pay for BiDil, any increase in prescription costs due to the drug would have been largely socialized rather than borne by African Americans alone.

More fundamentally, from the patient perspective, BiDil would be just a tiny part of a much larger burden. Most people are diagnosed with heart failure during a hospitalization event, and the debt burden of hospitalization is much more catastrophic than the burden of paying for a drug, even at BiDil's relatively high sticker price of $10 per day—and of course almost no patients pay the sticker price. Because A-HeFT suggested that patients taking BiDil would have fewer hospitalizations, BiDil would be more likely to lead to patients having lower medical care costs rather than higher ones. Although generic equivalents could of course lower costs further still, the far larger savings step would be in avoiding hospitalization—a fact that is obscured when analysts take pill prices out of context.

We should also bear in mind that heart failure itself is expensive. The disease is quite different from the asymptomatic conditions of risk, such as high cholesterol, that have been such a prominent part of Big Pharma's profitability.[45] People with heart failure have shortness of breath and fatigue, first with exertion, later with minor activity, and finally even at rest, so their ability to work is compromised. BiDil is just one of the perhaps eight or twelve drugs in their overall daily regimen. African Americans already had the highest rate of medical debt of any demographic group before the arrival of BiDil.[46] Applying abstract ethical principles to this drug in isolation is too limited an approach; it demands instead a "contextual bioethics" that is attentive to "structural limits and social complexities" in which patients navigate an onerous illness.[47] On both a broad historical trajectory and in many individual patients' lives, African American indebtedness resulting from medical costs precedes the existence of the poster child of race-based medicine, and there is a commodity fetishism in the fantasy that one somewhat expensive medicine can encapsulate this indebtedness. This framing obscures the scale and the magnitude of the costs of racially stratified medical care that extend beyond this or indeed any pill. There are a few pharmaceutical regimens that are exceptions to this rule, most notably many cancer treatments, in which the drugs themselves might be as expensive as hospitalization. But in the case of heart failure for self-identified Black patients, to the extent that they endure a debt burden for health care, the cost of BiDil is relatively trivial.

Thus, the cost of this pill is not necessarily the right focal point for our critical attention. The tangibility of a pill makes it a particularly appealing object for broader compelling critiques of race and medicine, but it can be misleading to foreground this object. The entire medical system is racially stratified, and we need to pay attention to what Alondra Nelson characterizes as the simultaneous undertreatment and overexposure to medical harms.[48] A disproportionate share of analytical attention has gone to (so far essentially unsuccessful) efforts to profit from race-based medicine, and to a lesser extent race-based denial of care, even though over a century of literature on the social determinants of health has shown us that race-based exposure to stress, poverty, incarceration, pollution, and other broader social phenomena are much more important in shaping embodied inequalities. In this sense, race-based pharmaceuticals are extremely minor issues.

The notion that a pill might be the solution to race-based inequality in health is resonant with the bioexpectations that Peter Redfield has described with respect to humanitarian medicine: the idea that cleverly designed technologies could be the solution to humanitarian crises.[49] Yet there are also important differences, which might help us understand

BiDil's failure to reach its markets. Redfield's examples—such as the "peepoo" that manages human excrement without water—are what he defines as "minimalist technologies" that are designed to accomplish their goals without any infrastructure. In contrast, BiDil only works as an adjunct to a highly intensive medical regimen. It is not necessarily a maximalist technology—which might be something like a neonatal intensive care unit or an organ transplantation unit—but BiDil certainly presumes the existence of health care infrastructure. The idea that a single pill could significantly affect not just the lives of particular patients at particular times but also racial inequality more broadly is part of a larger tendency to give undue analytical attention to technological objects. This is true not only when its proponents frame it as a solution to excessive burden of disease but also when its critics frame it as the locus of financial burden.

There are additional layers of compensation relations surrounding BiDil that are worthy of attention. One of the most compelling articulations of obligation in the discursive space around BiDil was the slogan of the ABC: "Children should know their grandparents." This is an individual imperative: grandparents should care for their health not only for their own sake but also for that of their families and communities. But it is also a social imperative: we should create a world in which children can know their grandparents. Among all of these compensation relations, this one is very much alive. The company owes its shareholders, but when the company goes bankrupt, they lose their investment. During the time of the trial, ABC and NitroMed had a reciprocal obligation: performing the trial in exchange for data to lead to an approvable drug; sponsorship in exchange for good will. However, once the trial is over, that compensation relation is closed. NitroMed is no more, whereas the ABC lives on. The ABC owes Black patients, and that does continue. Unlike the relationship with the pharmaceutical company or the particular FDA panel that approved BiDil, that relationship is not closed. For members of the ABC, the reality that drugs work for those who are able to access them will continue to resonate until the promise of access to health care and improved health outcomes becomes a reality for all Americans.

The term "race-based medicine" is often thought of as the development of race-specific pills, but we might instead see it as an entire system of care and its denial. Doing so sheds light on the limited critiques leveled at BiDil and its potential monetary costs to individuals rather than seeing it as a marginal element of the costs that a racialized system of care imposes on racialized populations and our society as a whole. Focusing on BiDil's failed marketing and distribution campaigns reveals both the limitations of the promise of particular pills, as well as the places that the compensation relations that move drugs to and through markets can break down. The specific actors, their relations, and the associated power dynamics involved in these breakdowns are in turn affected by, and affect, the broader racially stratified society.

BiDil in Context

In 2004, just as I was starting to explore the topic of race and heart disease, I attended my first of several conferences of the International Society for Hypertension in Blacks.[50] Sitting around the lunch table in that Detroit hotel meeting space making small talk, one attendee asked another if she was presenting anything. She said yes, she had a poster about a multidrug regimen for resistant hypertension. Asked whether it worked, she said, "In patients with prescription-coverage health insurance, it works great."

In the setting of this conference, this half joke pointed to one aspect of the context of racialized health care in the United States: the uneven burden of disease is exacerbated by unequal access to medical treatment, including pharmaceuticals. An unstated assumption that undergirds clinical trial results—that drugs work in patients who have access to the drugs—turns out to be problematic, particularly in racialized populations in the United States. Unimpeded access to pharmaceuticals is a key structural difference between African Americans in clinical trials and African Americans in the broader health care system.

The question of access to pharmaceuticals is not a simple or innocent one. The health disparities that contribute to the need for pharmaceuticals are fundamentally the result of living in a racially stratified society, and pharmaceuticals alone are only a small part of health care. Pharmaceutical companies have their vested financial interests, and other actors in the context of commodified health care are not disinterested either. Yet if we keep the question of access to medicines at the forefront, we can see that pharmaceuticals are not alternatives to social justice generally or to equitable treatment of African Americans in particular, but high-stakes components of these broader struggles.

When the doctor at the conference articulated access to insurance with prescription drug coverage as a determinant of a pharmaceutical protocol's efficacy, she incorporated the social into a biomedical discourse. The insight here is that although market-based distribution of drugs does not figure in clinical trials, it does shape the contours of pharmaceuticals' actually existing efficacy. Outrage over BiDil's racial indication spurred many righteous calls to focus on the social causes of disparities and to reject molecular ones, but the distribution of pharmaceuticals demonstrates a pathway by which social inequalities become molecular. In trials, BiDil was an impressive success, addressing a major health problem experienced by African Americans. Yet outside of the context of the drug trial, African American communities have not seen a dramatic result. A general medicalization critique of the limits of technological fixes for social problems is not sufficient.[51] Broken compensation relations are an important reason that the products of clinical trials cannot solve health disparities.

Notes

1. Troy Duster, "Race and Reification in Science," *Science* 307 (February 18, 2005): 1050–51; Pamela Sankar and Jonathan Kahn, "BiDil: Race Medicine or Race Marketing?," *Health Affairs,* suppl. Web Exclusive (2005): W5-455–63.

2. Brady Huggett, "BiDil Flops," *Nature Biotechnology* 26 (2008): 252.

3. See Ann H. Kelly and P. Wenzel Geissler, "Investigating the Ethics and Economics of Medical Experimentation," in *The Value of Transnational Medical Research: Labour, Participation and Care* (London: Routledge, 2012), 1–12.

4. See, e.g., Jonathan Kahn, *Race in a Bottle: The Story of BiDil and Racialized Medicine in a Post-genomic Age* (New York: Columbia University Press, 2012); Dorothy Roberts, "Color-Coded Pills," in *Fatal Invention: How Science, Politics, and Big Business Re-create Race in the Twenty-First Century* (New York: New Press, 2011): 168–201.

5. Kahn, *Race in a Bottle.*

6. Anne L. Taylor, Susan Ziesche, Clyde Yancy, et al., for the African-American Heart Failure Trial Investigators, "Combination of Isosorbide Dinitrate and Hydralazine in Blacks with Heart Failure," *New England Journal of Medicine* 351 (2004): 2049–57.

7. Sankar and Kahn, "BiDil."

8. Huggett, "BiDil Flops."

9. Sheldon Krimsky, "The Short Life of a Race Drug," *Lancet* 379, no. 9811 (2012): 114–15; Laurence J. Downey, "BiDil: Alive and Kicking," *Lancet* 379, no. 9829 (2012): 1876.

10. See Anne Pollock, "Transforming the Critique of Big Pharma," *BioSocieties* 6, no. 1 (2011): 106–18; Anne Pollock and David S. Jones, "Coronary Artery Disease and the Contours of Pharmaceuticalization," *Social Science and Medicine* 131 (2015): 250–71.

11. Mark Jewell, "Drug Maker Breaking New Ground with Grassroots Marketing of BiDil," *Target Market News,* April 11, 2006, http://targetmarketnews.com/. See also Britt M. Russert and Charmaine D. Royal, "Grassroots Marketing

in a Global Era: More Lessons from BiDil," *Journal of Law, Medicine, and Ethics* 39, no. 1 (2011): 79–90.

12. In 2012, the pharmaceutical industry spent $27 billion on promoting drugs, of which $24 billion went to advertising to physicians and $3 billion went to advertising to consumers. Pew Charitable Trusts, "Fact Sheet: Persuading the Prescribers: Pharmaceutical Industry Marketing and Its Influence on Physicians and Patients," November 11, 2013, http://www.pewtrusts.org/.

13. Chamika Hawkins-Taylor and Angeline M. Carlson, "Communication Strategies Must Be Tailored to a Medication's Targeted Population: Lessons from the Case of BiDil," *American Health and Drug Benefits* 6, no. 7 (2013): 401–12, fig. 2, http://www.ahdbonline.com/.

14. "Vigilante Company Profile," *Yahoo Finance*, archived at https://www.glassdoor.com.au/Overview/Working-at-Vigilante-EI_IE13851.11,20.htm.

15. "Publicis Groupe's Vigilante Top Executive Leaves to Form Own Shop," *PR Newswire*, April 12, 2010, http://www.prnewswire.com/.

16. The community outreach on BiDil was underwhelming even at the time, and those efforts left only a small footprint on the Web. When I searched the Internet in 2013, I was only able to find a single image of grassroots outreach of BiDil in practice, part of an Associated Press article: Mark Jewell, "Grassroots Marketing Brings a Pill to Its People," *Augusta Chronicle*, April 14, 2006 http://chronicle.augusta.com/.

17. Hawkins-Taylor and Carlson, "Communication Strategies."

18. This hierarchy of how modes of access—whether through elite specialists or through time-pressed practitioners serving poorer patients—shapes how patients relate to pharmaceuticals has been thoughtfully discussed by Emily Martin, "The Pharmaceutical Person," *BioSocieties* 1 (2006): 276.

19. Joy V. Fuqua, *Prescription TV: Therapeutic Discourse in the Hospital and the Home* (Durham, N.C.: Duke University Press, 2012): 100.

20. As of June 2, 2014, the coupon had been replaced by a $25 copay coupon, and as of December 15, 2016, the coupon is no longer available, replaced by a "Patient Direct Savings Program" with a $35 copay (https://www.bidil.com/).

21. Susan Cleary, Steve Birch, Natsayi Chimbindi, Sheetal Silal, and Di McIntyre, "Investigating the Affordability of Key Health Services in South Africa," *Social Science and Medicine* 80 (2013): 37–46; Ari Samsky, "'Since We Are Taking the Drugs': Labor and Value in Two International Drug Programs," *Journal of Cultural Economy* 4, no. 1 (2011): 27–43.

22. Emily Cohn, "Obamacare Has Drastically Cut the Uninsured Rate for Blacks, Hispanics," *Huffington Post,* June 5, 2014, http://huffingtonpost.com/.

23. David B. Nash, "Pharma Value," *American Health and Drug Benefits* 6, no. 8 (2013): 448–49.

24. David Grande, "The Cost of Drug Coupons," *Journal of the American Medical Association* 307, no. 22 (2012): 2375–76.

25. Stefan Ecks, "Global Pharmaceutical Markets and Corporate Citizenship: The Case of Novartis' Anti-cancer Drug Glivec," *BioSocieties* 3 (2008): 165–81.
26. Jeremy A. Greene, *Generic: The Unbranding of Modern Medicine* (Baltimore, Md.: Johns Hopkins University Press, 2014).
27. Craig M. Douglas, "NitroMed Agrees to be Sold for $36M," *Boston Business Journal,* June 30, 2009, http://www.bizjournals.com/.
28. Stephanie Saul, "FDA Approves a Heart Drug for African-Americans," *New York Times,* June 24, 2005, http://www.nytimes.com/.
29. Keith J. Winstein, "NAACP Presses on Heart Drug," *Wall Street Journal,* January 25, 2007, http://online.wsj.com/.
30. See Anne Pollock, *Medicating Race: Heart Disease and Durable Preoccupations with Difference* (Durham, N.C.: Duke University Press, 2012).
31. See "FDA User Fees: Current Measures Not Sufficient for Evaluating Effect on Public Health," *U.S. Government Accountability Office,* July 22, 1994, PEMD-94-26, http://www.gao.gov/.
32. U.S. Food and Drug Administration, Center for Biologics Evaluation and Research, *Performance Report to the President and Congress for the Prescription Drug User Fee Act,* fiscal year 2005, http://www.fda.gov/downloads/AboutFDA/ReportsManualsForms/Reports/UserFeeReports/PerformanceReports/ucm095108.pdf.
33. Department of Health and Human Services, Food and Drug Administration, Center for Drug Evaluation and Research, Cardiovascular and Renal Drugs Advisory Committee, "BiDil Open Public Hearing," transcript, vol. 2, June 16, 2005, http://www.fda.gov/ohrms/dockets/ac/05/transcripts/2005-4145T2.pdf, 203.
34. Ibid., 208.
35. Adriana Petryna, *Life Exposed: Biological Citizens after Chernobyl* (Princeton, N.J.: Princeton University Press, 2002), 6.
36. Jonathan Xavier Inda, "Materializing Hope: Racial Bodies, Suffering Bodies, and Biological Citizenship," in *Corpus: an Interdisciplinary Reader on Bodies and Knowledge,* ed. Monica Casper and Paisley Currah (New York: Palgrave Macmillan, 2011).
37. U.S. Food and Drug Administration, "BiDil Open Public Hearing," 307–8.
38. Ibid., 309.
39. See Ruha Benjamin, "Organized Ambivalence: When Sickle Cell Disease and Stem Cell Research Converge," *Ethnicity and Health* 16, no. 4–5 (2011): 447–63.
40. Winstein, "NAACP Presses on Heart Drug."
41. Daniel J. Pompeo and Richard A. Samp, "Petition of Washington Legal Foundation to the Centers for Medicare and Medicaid Services . . . Concerning Coverage for BiDil under Federal Health Care Programs," August 7, 2008, http://www.wlf.org/upload/BIDIL.pdf, 10.
42. Jonathan Xavier Inda, *Racial Prescriptions: Pharmaceuticals, Difference, and the Politics of Life* (London: Ashgate, 2014), 106.

43. Ibid.

44. Duana Fullwiley, "The Molecularization of Race: Institutionalizing Human Difference in Pharmacogenetics Practice," *Science as Culture* 16, no. 1 (2007): 2.

45. Joseph Dumit, *Drugs for Life: How Pharmaceutical Companies Define Our Health* (Durham, N.C.: Duke University Press, 2012); Jeremy Greene, *Prescribing by Numbers: Drugs and the Definition of Disease* (Baltimore, Md.: Johns Hopkins University Press, 2006).

46. Michelle M. Doty and Alyssa L. Holmgren, "Health Care Disconnect: Gaps in Coverage and Care for Minority Adults," *Commonwealth Fund* 21 (2006): 1–12.

47. These terms are drawn from Jennifer S. Singh's work on the very different disease context of autism. Singh, "Narratives of Participation in Autism Genetics Research," *Science, Technology, and Human Values* 40, no. 2 (2015): 237.

48. Alondra Nelson, *Body and Soul: The Black Panther Party and the Fight against Medical Discrimination* (Minneapolis: University of Minnesota Press, 2011).

49. Peter Redfield, "Bioexpectations: Life Technologies as Humanitarian Goods," *Public Culture* 24, no. 1 (2012): 157–84.

50. The 2004 annual conference of the International Society for Hypertension in Blacks was held at the Detroit Marriott Renaissance Center, June 13–16, 2004.

51. See Scott Vrecko, "Global and Everyday Matters of Consumption: On the Productive Assemblage of Pharmaceuticals and Obesity," *Theory and Society* 39 (2010): 555–73, esp. 570–71.

II
RACE-BASED MEDICINE
AND INDEBTEDNESS

5

The Meaning of Health Disparities

CATHERINE BLISS

In the late 1980s, when genetic scientists embarked upon the study of genomics (the science of DNA sequences), the concept of health disparities was itself emerging from public health debates over racial and gender inequality. The U.S. government believed that it was morally indebted to racial minorities for years of neglect and that research targeted to minority experiences would begin to identify ways to alleviate racial inequality. At this time, the study of DNA sequences and racial inequality were separate endeavors. Early health disparities experts struggled to characterize the relationship between socioeconomic status, experiences of racial discrimination, institutionalized racism, and social processes of categorization and identification that shape health outcomes, while genomic pioneers set about the task of mapping the human genome. Policy makers and experts believed that payback for racial inequality required economic and political means targeted to advance the social standing of minorities, while the study of genes in tandem required a suspension of social inquiries and thought. DNA science worked to remain color-blind, or blind of race and its relationship to genes and health.

Yet as governmental and public health agencies moved forward with race-targeted research, this instantiated a policy that mandated all federally funded research to sample by race—research focused on biological health factors as well as social health factors. With its promise to revolutionize health care through personalized medicine, genomics would come to carry the banner of race-focused medicine.

Today, the very genomic sciences that once stood outside of public debates over the meaning of health disparities are leading governmental public health efforts in this domain. In the United States, the federal public health establishment grants genomic research the greatest amount of research dollars to study health disparities, and as a result, health disparities are increasingly studied in genomic terms that ignore economic and political factors, despite decades of research implicating these factors as the primary determinants of racial health disparities. Redress has been reconceived in scientific terms that stop short of changing the social relations that perpetuate racial inequality. In its efforts to pursue and maintain funding, genomics has commandeered U.S. government efforts to bring attention to minority communities and racial health disparities. In the process, notions of race and health disparities have been increasingly biologized, and redress for social inequality has been reenvisioned in the form of pills and diagnostics.

Yet moral indebtedness cannot be rectified through the medicalization of structural disadvantage. Race and health disparities must be understood as social entities, and they must be addressed through systemic structural change to health care, neighborhoods, and other aspects of the built environment. Scientists responsible for seminal genome projects, who have faced pressure from the U.S. public health establishment and an array of experts on health disparities, now prioritize race-targeted research, minority recruitment, and analysis of genomic health disparities. As a result, large-scale sequencing projects, pharmaceuticals, and postgenomic research have become ever more racialized, while race has taken on an irrevocably genomic imprimatur at the expense of its former social characterization.

I begin with an examination of the ways in which research inclusion by race came to be the predominant biomedical solution to solving the moral crisis of racial inequality. I show how scientists and policy makers framed genomic inclusion as the best redress for government neglect of minority communities. I then discuss the ways in which genome projects and clinical trials appropriated the debt problem, offering racialized medicine as the new gold standard in racial redress. I conclude by examining the problematic ethical implications of genomics as redress, including its negligence and obfuscation of economic and political understandings of race and health. I caution that this approach ensures that scientific indebtedness will continue to eclipse social indebtedness unless sociological factors are again put at the center of research.

It is worth nothing that the concept of debt that I write about focuses less on the traditional notion of the word and its emphasis on owing money, goods, and services. Instead, I advance a concept of debt that rests on a more capacious view of social obligation, one that captures the structural factors involved in redressing social neglect. In the case of race, an array of advocates, activists, and policy makers have petitioned for monetary redress (e.g., slavery reparations in the case of African Americans and territorial reparations in the case of Native Americans) for the centuries of institutionalized racism that have led to the health inequalities we see today. While the U.S. government acknowledges its indebtedness to minority communities, it has not embraced redress in terms of money, goods, or services as a solution.

Transformations in Genome Projects

Looking back at the advent of genomic research, it is evident that there was no framework for interpreting the meaning of health disparities and no genomic entertainment of racial analysis or health disparities analysis at the start of the genome era. When the National Institutes of Health (NIH), the Department of Energy, and the world's leading human geneticists launched the Human Genome Project in 1986, scientists took no notice of race or health disparities. Planning meeting minutes generated by a range of national, international, and supranational public health divisions, including project management branches, advisory councils, and financial departments, show none of the informal conversation on race that later colored project endeavors. At the level of DNA sampling and sequencing, Human Genome Project scientists did not consider DNA in population terms. In fact, they made a copy of all the DNA in one human organism by sequencing immortalized cell lines of convenience from the Centre d'Etude du Polymorphisme Humain, which were known to primarily derive from a set of European American donors from Utah.[1]

In the wider culture, debates raged over the need to acknowledge racial inequality. In response, social and political analysts from a variety of fields advanced a color-blind framework in which racial justice would be brought about by refusing to see race.[2] This era exhibited a one-size-fits-all framework, wherein research populations were assumed to be biomedically equal and one subject's biomaterial could stand in for another's.[3] Protecting so-called vulnerable populations—that is, racial minorities with significant histories of mistreatment in biomedicine and public health—meant treating them the same as Whites. Indeed, postwar geneticists working in the shadow of eugenics worked to cleanse popular culture of the term "race" by transferring it to the scientific domain.[4] By the start of the Human Genome Project, researchers tried equally hard to exorcise the term from genetics.

Even as the Human Genome Project established its Ethical, Legal, and Social Issues branch in 1990, scientists did not mention race.[5] The Human Genome Project expanded its second Five Year Plan's goals to "foster greater acceptance of human genetic variation" and to "enhance and expand public and professional education that is sensitive to sociocultural and psychological issues." However, it did not discuss variation or sociocultural issues in terms of race.[6]

Still, behind closed doors, public health officials were working hard to integrate the Office of Management and Budget's Directive No. 15, a standard set of racial classifications of White, Black, American Indian and Alaska Native, and Asian or Pacific Islander mandated to report inclusion and participation in existing and emerging programs.[7] Congress had issued Directive No. 15 in the late 1970s, after years of deliberation over how to structure a post–Civil Rights Act and post–Voting Rights Act system of governance that could repay the U.S. government's debt to minorities. However, it took the better part of the following decade to institute federal standards into biomedicine.[8] By 1990, the U.S. government had established minority and women's task forces and offices for special populations health across the Department of Health and Human Services (HHS), and underserved populations and minority health were focal interests of the surgeon general's office and the entire public health department. In fact, the office's 1990 decennial Healthy People statement claimed that the new direction in American public health would be to "increase the span of healthy life," "achieve access to preventive services," and "reduce health disparities . . . among all Americans."[9]

The color-blind, one-size-fits-all framework began to turn in earnest the year that the NIH issued the Revitalization Act of 1993. This statute set guidelines for the surveillance and inclusion of women and racial minorities in all research funded by the NIH.[10] The Centers for Disease Control and Prevention simultaneously issued the "Use of Race and Ethnicity in Public Health Surveillance," a statement affirming Directive No. 15's import to public health.[11] Now the agencies responsible for the majority of genomics funding worldwide were coming under the policy to use U.S. federal race classifications. Tides were turning toward a race-conscious framework in which scientists would come to play a key role.

As the Human Genome Project refined its sampling and sequencing methods, another genome project got underway. The Human Genome Diversity Project was devised as a corollary genome project that would focus on the now pressing matter of diversity. In fact, the Human Genome Diversity Project banked its reputation as the first global project to capture all the human diversity in the world. At its opening, the project received support from Human Genome Project officials, who agreed that there was a dire need for a genome project focused on characterizing human diversity. However, the project refused to use Directive No. 15 categories to structure its research.[12] Project leaders who had only recently begun removing the word "race" from their publications were taken aback at the directive to reinstitute racial categories. Despite further sponsorship from the Department of Energy, the National Science Foundation, the National Institute of General Medical Sciences, and the National Human Genome Research Center, the project's plan to ignore race drew criticism from government and lay advocates.[13]

Eventually project planners got on board with the new framework and began discussing racial sampling strategies with minority scientists and health advocates.[14] When, in 1995, the HHS ordered the National Research Council to investigate the Human Genome Diversity Project's plans for recruiting vulnerable populations, the project leaders responded with a public declaration that the project would "combat the scourge of racism" in terms relevant to U.S. racial minorities and the U.S. government's social, moral, and political debt to them.[15] Under threat of dissolution, planners changed the project's recruitment policy to include members of U.S. minority groups following Directive No. 15 guidelines. Though the project failed to convince organizations such as the National Research Council that it would be able to protect its minority research subjects, it set a precedent for the rest of the field that race and the debt of health inequality mattered.[16]

The shift toward a framework that would allow for a genomic investigation of race and health disparities was equally felt in the broader institutions of health governance that were increasingly focusing efforts on genomics. In 1996, the Department of Energy and National Human Genome Research Center, two agencies that had formerly ignored women and minority issues, issued a new mandate to include women in genetic research. This echoed Directive No. 15's policy claiming that, though there was not sufficient biological evidence that men and women (in this case, male and female autosomal chromosomes) could not stand in for one another, the social history of female exclusion was enough of an issue to warrant new recruitment protocols.[17] Agreement was shared by all agencies that the government's obligation to redress inequality was enough to restructure and marshal the nation's most eminent scientific resources.

The NIH's Ethical, Legal, and Social Issues branch also embarked on policy making for the recruitment of racial minorities in the guise of conferences on minority community intervention. When Congress reissued Directive No. 15 the following year, in hopes of securing greater compliance in the HHS and its subagencies, such as the U.S. Food and Drug Administration (FDA), the National Human Genome Research Center was elevated to the status of a NIH institute. The FDA issued a new policy that mandated researchers to compare drug dose and efficacy in racial groups, while the National Human Genome Research Institute moved to construct a genome project entirely structured by race. These agencies fought to establish themselves as the leading supporters of race-focused research. They opened up a host of race-targeted funding mechanisms that could bring genomics to bear on racial redress.

The Polymorphism Discovery Project utilized Directive No. 15 classifications to sample and then distribute DNA collections for use in research.[18] As this two-year project came to a close, and as the Human Genome Project also prepared to conclude, the National Human Genome Research Institute released a new goal for exploring "how socioeconomic factors and concepts of race and ethnicity influence the use, understanding, and interpretation of genetic information, the utilization of genetic services, and the development of policy."[19] The NIH simultaneously formulated its first funding mechanism dedicated to understanding the social factors involved with race, such as perceptions and identities. "Concepts of Race, Ethnicity, and Culture: Examination of the Ways in Which the Discovery of DNA Polymorphisms May Interact with Current Concepts of Race, Ethnicity and Culture" sponsored investigator projects on race, but it also fostered the creation of an in-house interdisciplinary Race and Genetics Working Group. Meanwhile, similar policy-making councils were assembled in the HHS in order to ensure that understanding race would be a centerpiece of genomics.

Thus, at the turn of the century, as the Human Genome Project celebrated its successful publication of a draft map on Capitol Hill and the HHS prepared a new set of decennial health goals, the paradigm shift was nearly complete. Racial classifications à la Directive No. 15 were instated across the field of genomics, and genome projects were attuned to redressing racial inequality. As race permeated and restructured basic research, genomic science was remade in ways that could begin to repay the U.S. government's moral debt to minority communities.

The Rise of Race-based Genomic Medicine

New racial matters of concern led scientists, policy makers, and the public to debate whether genomic medicine should be race based. Following the FDA's mandate to compare pharmacokinetics and pharmacodynamics by

THE MEANING OF HEALTH DISPARITIES 113

race in all clinical trials, drug developers working in the emerging research area of pharmacogenomics began insisting on the inclusion of minority subjects in research as a way to generate personalized medicine for groups previously neglected. Genaissance Pharmaceuticals' Gualberto Ruaño celebrated the potential for pharmacogenomics to transform biomedicine by arguing that genomics would demonstrate efficacy "in small cohorts of a few hundred patients compared to 3,000 or 5,000."[20] Trial scientists espoused race–gender variation in drug metabolism and clinical trials research reports, simultaneously realizing and propagating the FDA's race-comparative approach.

In 2001, the makers of BiDil, the fixed-dose combination of a generic antihypertensive and vasodilator generated solely for use in people of African descent, further paved the way for race-specific pharmacogenomic clinical trials when they conducted a Blacks-only clinical trial and a post hoc racial analysis of their prior trials.[21] The scientific community accepted their results of differential racial outcomes as proof of some underlying genetic variation by race. For example, in the pages of the *New England Journal of Medicine,* where post hoc analyses were published, two editorials spun a debate over the merits of racial pharmacogenomics off the BiDil results.[22] Though these editorials did not agree about the merits of race-based medicine, they echoed the study's authors in calling for more pharmacogenomics research into minority health and a proactive inclusion of minorities in health sciences and biomedicine.

The developing approach to racial redress was further encapsulated in the 2001 inaugural issue of the *Pharmacogenomics Journal,* which hosted a debate over race-based medicine wherein a diverse array of scientists agreed that inclusion of minorities was the only way to protect their interests in leading the U.S. government's racial redress charge. These representatives of the burgeoning genomic community defined health rights in terms of access to genomic therapies; they therefore sought ways to reconceptualize race differently than prior genetic deterministic models. Powerful racial advocacy organizations that had long fought for health rights using radical reconceptualizations of race and health[23] also began defining equality in terms of access to personalized medicine. Leading African American advocacy groups, such as the NAACP, the National Medical Association, and the Association of Black Cardiologists, supported BiDil's makers' intent to conduct a Blacks-only clinical trial. Scientists and advocates exchanged tropes of identity politics, further crystallizing the normative frameworks that required a framework useful for spotlighting the genetic and social aspects of race. As Jay Cohn, BiDil's principal scientist and patent holder, summed it up, "Here we have the black community accepting the concept that African Americans need to be studied as a group, and then we have the science community claiming that race is dead. . . . It seems to me absolutely ludicrous to suggest that this prominent characteristic that we all recognize when we look at people should not be looked at."[24] The mélange of scientists, policy makers, and public representatives that offered BiDil as a solution to color-blindness and one-size-fits-all medicine offered the nascent genomics community a new way of approaching intractable issues of race. When the National Human Genome Research Institute opened talks for a new international genome project, genomic leaders made it clear that race would be a front and center issue. Eric Lander, a foundational planner of the Human Genome Project who would chair the new project's Methods Group, argued, "We must make sure the information is not used to stigmatize populations. But we have an affirmative responsibility to ensure that what is learned will be useful for all populations. If we shy away and don't record the data for certain populations, we can't be sure to serve those populations medically."[25] Again, race-conscious research and clinical trial protocols were lauded as the only way to ensure repayment of the debt owed these communities—nothing short of equal opportunity for racial minorities. The newly minted International HapMap Project, a project set to sequence genomic haplotypes in world populations, settled on Directive No. 15 relevant study populations "representing several racial groups,"[26] specifically "African, Asian, and Caucasian chromosomes," despite acknowledging that racial categories were socially constructed and had no basis in biology.[27] Indeed, the International HapMap Project's official introductory article in *Nature* articulated the incoming redress approach. It interpreted the project's value in terms of its ability to attain biological, global representation and social, racial inclusivity.[28] Vague characterizations of the links between genetic variation and social inequality would condition all future communiqués.

As the International HapMap Project rolled out, two project scientists at Howard University proposed the first race-specific genome-sequencing project. This African American Diversity Project promised to extend cutting-edge, personalized medicine to African Americans by including them in basic sequencing groundwork. In the language of access popular among identity-based organizations, cofounder Charles Rotimi stated: "If you want your clothes to fit, you'd better go to the tailor to be measured."[29] Cofounder Georgia Dunston further argued that participation was the only way to secure coverage of Black American health issues.[30]

Taking a truly redress-focused tack, the project's leaders claimed that the race-specific biobank would be the first project to study, and seek therapeutic solutions to, the genomic health effects of racism. Though the planners did not detail how they would incorporate social measures of race, their expressed intent set a tone for what the scientific community and its public health collaborators conceived as possible. In particular, their claims rallied scientists working in the emerging field of translational genomics. For example, members of the NIH Pharmacogenomics Research Network and a team of translational scientists at Stanford University published op-eds calling for genomic analyses of race. "There is great validity in racial/ethnic self-categorizations, both from the research and public policy points of view," wrote Center for Pharmacogenomics director Neil Risch and colleagues.[31]

In 2004, BiDil's makers reported the successful results of the drug's final clinical trial. Months before, trial scientists had abruptly put an end to the trial when they witnessed a 43 percent relative one-year mortality decrease in the self-identified Black subjects who had taken the drug. Within months, the FDA approved the drug for market. Though neither the pharmacogenomic nor the pharmacokinetic and pharmacodynamics mechanisms of the drug were determined,[32] scientists, policy makers, and public representatives alike framed the drug as a frontline weapon in the fight against racial health disparities and inequality.[33]

Since BiDil's approval, there has been an upsurge of support from U.S. funding and regulatory agencies, health justice groups, and community representatives for race-based medicine. More race-based therapies have been patented and brought to market,[34] such as the lung cancer drug Iressa for Asians and the antihypertensive Bystolic for Mexicans. Buoyed by these successes, the U.S. Patent Office has called for new patent applications to take race into consideration.[35] Both the American College of Medical Genetics and the FDA have similarly called for the testing of drug response by race in blockbusters, or drugs that generate over $1 billion in revenue per year. Meanwhile, health rights activists and racial justice advocates have joined the boards of pharmaceutical companies designing race-based therapies,[36] thereby legitimizing the framework within nongovernmental organizations. Finally, bioethicists interested in the growing genomic divide have petitioned for race-based drugs that can be used in underserved populations in the Global South, including unsuccessful chemical combinations that bioethicists argue may be resuscitated for underserved populations.[37] Together, these developments show that the health justice framework that promotes race-based medicine as a necessary shortcut to leveling the playing field via scientific redress is now securely an upstream part of research conceptualization and a downstream trope of social justice. Indeed, these developments have led to cuts in social determinants research and a spike in genomic funding for studying health disparities.

Race in Scientists' Terms

The normative and epistemic dimensions of this framework are best witnessed in scientists' own articulations. Genome scientists who have lead the move from DNA sequencing to functional analysis of genomes, including epigenomics and gene–environment research, have embodied the paradigm shift. In their coming to consciousness about race and its import for science, leading genomicists have transformed the landscape of research design and implementation worldwide.

It is first important to note that scientists' present-day criticisms of simplistic genetic characterizations of race have arisen in part from formal dialogues with experts on the sociology of race. Policy forums taking place since the mapping of the human genome, such as Ethical, Legal, and Social Issues branch-sponsored conferences, seminars, and councils, provided repeated opportunities for experts to advise genome scientists to eliminate the wanton use of social concepts of race in their research and to ask scientists to consider their role in promoting a specific set of racial relations. Experts entreated genomicists to think critically about the biology of racism: "It is not that *different* biological processes underlie disease formation in different races, but that different life experience activates physiological processes common to all, but less provoked in some."[38] They recommended that genome scientists take a systems biology approach to racial health disparities, wherein scientists would approach genes as subject to modulation from the environment.

This alternate approach was a direct response to color-blind, one-size-fits-all science; however, it was not a request to simply use racial classifications more frequently and consistently. In fact, policy advisors insisted on the rhetorical power of genomics in the wider society, with many petitioning for genomic scientists to only use Directive No. 15 classifications in studies that had anything to do with the biology of racial discrimination. As Troy Duster, a sociologist and member of numerous genome project councils, argued:

> Under some conditions, we need to conduct systematic investigation, guided by a body of theory, into the role of "race" (or ethnicity, or

religion) as an organizing force in social relations, and as a stratifying practice. Under other conditions, we will need to conduct systematic investigation, guided by a body of theory, into the role of the interaction of "race" (or ethnicity, or religion) however flawed as a biologically discrete and coherent taxonomic system, with feedback loops into the biological functioning of the human body; or with medical practice. The latter studies might include examination of the systematic administration of higher doses of x-rays to African Americans; the creation of genetic tests with high rates of sensitivity to some ethnic and racial groups, but low sensitivity to others; and the systematic treatment, or lack of it, with diagnostic and therapeutic interventions to "racialized" heart and cancer patients.[39]

Duster's approach suggested that scientists change their study aims and research variables to measure the biological effects of racist social structures, such as the higher prevalence of certain toxins in the body of racial minorities who live or work in unhealthy sites. This was indeed an argument to study racial health disparities and to deploy a gene–environment perspective that draws on an interdisciplinary set of knowledge. However, a gene–environment study to this effect would not begin examining the population-based frequencies of genetic variants until far after the systemic sociology of the disorder was understood.

The genome scientists most associated with these policy forums interpreted these messages as a call for gene–environmental approaches in genomics and an active program of investigation of race. For example, the Broad Institute's Mark Daly, a Pfizer Fellow in Computational Biology and creator of the influential GeneHunter program, echoed Duster's sentiments in a call for richer gene–environmental research design: "There are so many elements of epidemiologic data collection—collecting information about people's diets, upbringing, and so forth—that need greater attention, maybe greater technological advances so that we could bring some of those in as well." In an interview at the Broad, he discussed how to incorporate a panoply of social epidemiological measures into genomic models, with race being but one. He and others at the Broad espoused their vision for a genomic biostatistical revolution in health disparities research, emphasizing how its robust computational tools would benefit disparities research in all fields. However, Daly exhibited the fuzziness with which genome scientists approach the genomic and social factors attributed to race: "It is often difficult to distinguish whether one's genetic continent of origin is the risk factor or if it's simply the access to healthcare or how seriously your medical issues get taken by the medical establishment, depending on what your background is." Because the genomic vision of race is not guided by a theory and is in effect untheorized, it has not provided clear directions for researchers interested in conducting a gene–environment analysis that would apprehend health care and delivery disparities.

In further conversation, Daly maintained that genomic statistical models would better root out causes of disparities than other public health fields. Using his own research into inflammatory bowel disorder and Crohn disease in people of European descent as an example, he discussed the rise and fall of certain disorders with respect to the changing environment and standard of living. Yet though Daly was able to make a nuanced gene–environmental argument for the racial disparity in these disorders, he was not able to show proof of their environmental causes because no environmental research to that effect had been conducted. His expressed concerns show how the genomic racial redress framework operates to prioritize race and health disparities in the ranks of genetic science at the same time as it fails to produce significant alterations to the genomic mode of analysis. Scientists can pay lip service to social determinants of health without ever investigating those determinants or incorporating study of them into their research.

Comments from Georgia Dunston, the aforementioned founder of the African Genome Diversity Project and Founding Director of Howard University's National Human Genome Center, also bespeak the power and limitations of the genomic approach. In her office at Howard University's Cancer Hospital, she linked African American genomic health outcomes to racial identification and ascription, articulating the feedback loop that Duster highlighted: "What is the internal influence . . . for a person who, because of certain biological characteristics, perceives themself [sic] or their continuity or integrity as being threatened—whether it is getting a job, losing a job, getting insurance, losing insurance?" While Dunston's Genomic Research in African American Pedigrees Project has set out to create a representative reference database of African American DNA common health issues so that the diseases that African Americans face can be better understood, and while her current gene–environment study of asthma seeks to understand the relationship between racism-based social variance and genetic variance, it is not clear how the environment is better measured in such large-scale sequencing projects. Though Dunston and other genome scientists, especially those who self-identity as African American, as Dunston does, maintain an earnest interest in understanding the relationship between "discrimination, racism, and stressors" and health, research protocols show greater investment in genomic methods to the detriment of measures for the sociological context.

Perhaps the clearest example of the pitfalls of the genomic racial redress framework is the move to race-based genome projects. While the African Genome Diversity Project did not garner enough funding to launch, it was reformulated by Charles Rotimi when he took directorship of the NIH Intramural Center for Health Disparities Genomics, now known as the Center for Research on Genomics and Global Health. Rotimi, a genetic epidemiologist who was the delegate researcher to his native Nigeria in the International HapMap Project, had been working on institutionalizing a gene–environmental model in genomics and public health for some time. Rotimi had participated in Ethical, Legal, and Social Issues branch publications and National Human Genome Research Institute science advisory panels on race before founding the first center at the NIH that would entirely focus on the genomics of racial health disparities. In a meeting convened during the Center for Health Disparities Genomics' emergence, he explained how he envisioned the relationship between genes and the environment in his work:

> People who socialize together tend to eat things that are similar. . . . Even our culturation in terms of who goes out to do a 10K versus someone who stays in front of the TV, or if you notice, someone who sits around your kitchen and tell[s] stories. . . . Those have been passed on [through] health.
> So if you want to look at a disparity, you have to look at income. You have to look at education. You have to look at why is it that you find certain people more in jail than others. Why is it that certain people are in a certain business more than others? Why is it that certain people tend to live closer to dumps than others? You have to look at the social structures.

Despite successfully marshaling public health forces around the world to launch an international project dedicated to the genomics of the African diaspora—the Human Health and Heredity in Africa Project—none of these sociological measures has been included. In fact, the only nonphysiological environmental measure that has been implemented to date is that of urban versus rural dwelling.

Thus, the Human Health and Heredity in Africa Project has only served to enlarge support for the sequencing of people of African descent, and the use of those sequences in comparative studies with other racial groups. It has not encouraged a balanced gene–environmental approach in genomics and public health. The genomic approach to health disparities pulls resources for genome projects that promise to conduct in-house social epidemiological research, but only do so in narrow biological terms.

Gene–Environment Research as Payback

Since the turn of the millennium, public health research budgets worldwide have increasingly been directed toward research into gene–environment interactions and epigenetic and translational science. Amid these changes, in the United States, the HHS has deemed racial health disparities genomics a top funding priority.[40] In the interest of further institutionalizing gene–environment research into health disparities, the NIH has sponsored new funding mechanisms for research centers and laboratories across the country. In turn, it has propelled the genomic racial redress framework into ever-new arenas and research frameworks while forging societal interests in it across a wider range of social contexts.

Institutionalization began in 2003, when the NIH introduced an institutional award for Centers for Population Health and Health Disparities. In five years, five centers were funded, and ten more had been scheduled for funding.[41] The award announcement expressed a gene–environment approach to health disparities in its intent "to explain how the social and built environments impact biological processes."[42] Yet the award's target variables were "epigenetic modifications, gene expression, endocrine function, inflammation, tumor growth, and cancer-related health outcomes,"[43] not neighborhood effects and social stratification.

That same year, the National Human Genome Research Institute, the Department of Energy, and the National Institute for Child Health and Human Development also issued an institutional award for Centers of Excellence in Ethical, Social, and Legal Issues Research. This interinstitute, interorganization national public health alliance intended for funded institutions to serve as hubs of gene–environment health justice research. The award announcement specifically called for proposers to partner with minority institutions, especially race-based associations and historically Black universities. As the National Human Genome Research Institute exclaimed in its accompanying 2004–8 Health Disparities Plan:

> Special emphasis will be placed on access to information, informed consent, community attitudes toward genetic research; emphasis will also be placed on the development of methods to optimize informed decision-making regarding participation in genetic research and use of the knowledge gained through this research. It is hoped that the

research supported by this initiative will increase information available to investigators that will help them to design future genetic research in a way that will more successfully involve minority communities.[44]

In other words, though funding would be equally available to research on the sociological dimensions of race, funders intended to support research that would facilitate the acceptance and implementation of genetic research. Research inclusion and enrollment were the focus of these efforts of institutionalization. Thus, in its first round, the Centers of Excellence in Ethical, Social, and Legal Issues Research program went on to provide over $20 million in grants to study issues such as breast cancer and asthma in people of African descent. It has since continued to fund centers focused on gene–environment research into diabetes, prostate cancer, and sickle cell anemia in minority communities as a result of these disorders' overwhelming racial disparity.

Institutionalization has taken place within the public health establishment as well. Since 2007, agencies within the U.S. HHS have launched two federal research centers dedicated to health disparities gene–environment research. The first of these institutes is Rotimi's Center for Research on Genomics and Global Health. Again, this institute's focus is the genomics of diseases that contribute to health inequities affecting African Americans. The second of these institutes is the Centers for Disease Control and Prevention's Office of Public Health Genomics, the mission of which is "to convey the importance of engaging communities, investing in [community-based public research] and ensuring that social justice be central to public health genomics."[45] It deems race and gender stratification as a focal point of gene–environment inquiry. However, it remains to be seen whether sociological measures will be included in its research repertoire as the office's work unfolds.

Taken together, support for the institutionalization of research institutes framed with genomic goals still pales in comparison to the ways in which the genomic approach to repaying racial debts has rooted into the central administrative bodies of the American public health apparatus. The study of diseases that exhibit disparities by race lead the priority foci of innovation agendas of the suprainstitute, supradepartmental order. In the NIH, the largest funding opportunities in existence are the transinstitute mechanisms. In recent years, the NIH has announced that it will focus funding on gene–environment research, and that transinstitute proposals that include a health disparities component will be more competitive. The NIH Task Force on Obesity, for example, cites health disparities epigenetics and intrauterine interactions as it new aim; it thus encourages applications from those who are willing to conduct race-focused work. The NIH Common Fund, the organization's main suprainstitute division, has also stated its intent to prioritize research that has a dual gene–environment and racial health disparity focus. As it states, "Disadvantaged populations may experience greater exposure to [environmental] hazards and exhibit higher rates of disease incidence, morbidity and mortality. Understanding and modulating this risk in humans during critical windows of development offers the promise of primary prevention for many of these NCDs [noncommunicable diseases] and may result in reducing health disparities."[46] Most critical about this announcement is the fact that the Common Fund was established for the purpose of encouraging a gene–environment science revolution in the public health establishment, specifically through promoting a developmental biology approach to gene–environment research in noncommunicable chronic disease research. The Common Fund thus holds a monopoly over the resources that will guide the various institutes' transformations for years to come. Their appropriation of a genomic approach has a pyramid-like affect on all publicly funded research.

Indeed, the Common Fund has stipulated a gene–environment approach for the newest genome project and for the first-ever prospective cohort genome project, the Synthetic Cohort for the Analysis of Longitudinal Effects of Gene–Environment Interactions, in which characterization of the NIH's three focal diseases for health disparities gene–environment research—diabetes, hypertension, and prostate cancer—will be priority aims. Likewise, the Gene–Environment Initiative, initiated by the HHS in 2006,[47] and its National Human Genome Research Institute branch, GENEVA, has also focused on "pathways to disparities in health outcomes."[48] Yet as genomics-led gene–environment research becomes the mandate of President Barack Obama's Global Health Initiative and the mainstay of the NIH global health research, "small molecule screening, genomics of pathogens, and vaccine development"[49] will continue to trump "the systematic administration of higher doses of x-rays to African Americans; the creation of genetic tests with high rates of sensitivity to some ethnic and racial groups, but low sensitivity to others; and the systematic treatment, or lack of it, with diagnostic and therapeutic interventions to 'racialized' heart and cancer patients."[50] Thus far, funds have been awarded to genetic epidemiologists and genomicists. Social epidemiology has been all but absent from the picture, and sociology has been completely ignored. This framework thus promises to advance a genomic-heavy, sociology-light social justice program into the coming decades, the result of which will be further emphasis on pharmacological solutions and further neglect of the social determinants of health.

Conclusion

Since the advent of the genomic racial redress framework, the landscape of biomedicine and public health has been transformed into one dominated by a highly racialized postgenomic public health system, replete with racialized databases, protocols, and standards. Health disparities research budgets enlarge every year, and increasingly all publicly funded research is beholden to the racial impetus of racial redress. Yet expanding emphases on race have not rendered the social and built environment visible. Nor has any tangible form of repayment or redress been rendered to the subjects these programs were meant to help.

Researchers argue that the only way to produce equality is to study racial difference by relying on racial classifications. Yet a closer examination of the environmental or social components of their research shows there to be an extensive study of genetic factors and a minimal study of health behaviors. Moreover, researchers put no attention to the other social, economic, and political measures that once dominated conceptions of health disparities. Critical issues like transgenerational health effects, institutionalized forms of discrimination, and social environments are poorly understood.

What is most challenging about contesting the genomic approach is its fit with an increasingly geneticizing world. The health disparities genomics framework is increasingly a societal one, and one endemic to a range of social institutions beyond the halls of science. As I have shown, development of scientific redress is monopolized by a small community of scientific experts while being supported by a wide array of social groups to whom the government seeks to better serve. Yet for a truly equitable approach to biomedicine and public health, as well as for the study of human diversity, this imbalance in knowledge aims and production must be rectified.

In the meantime, as Duster has argued, unless race is theorized sociologically in studies, genomic researchers should refrain from adopting social classifications. So although genetic and social factors are inextricable, and although race has biological effects worth studying from a gene–environment perspective, the sociology of race must be unpacked before it is plugged into a study and research on social determinants of health should be prioritized. If "race, used as a stratifying practice, has produced what could be read as negative health practices,"[51] that process of stratification is what has yet to be explained. Scientific indebtedness must be rendered as social indebtedness, and health disparities recast with new meaning.

Notes

1. Catherine Bliss, *Race Decoded: The Genomic Fight for Social Justice* (Stanford, Calif.: Stanford University Press, 2012).

2. Michael Omi and Howard Winant, *Racial Formation in the United States: From the 1960s to the 1990s,* 2nd ed. (New York: Routledge, 1994).

3. Steven Epstein, *Inclusion: The Politics of Difference in Medical Research* (Chicago: University of Chicago Press, 2007).

4. Jenny Reardon, *Race to the Finish: Identity and Governance in an Age of Genomics* (Princeton, N.J.: Princeton University Press, 2005).

5. National Institutes of Health (NIH), "Understanding Our Genetic Inheritance: The U.S. Human Genome Project. The First Five Years: Fiscal Years 1991–1995," *Human Genome Project Information Archive, 1990–2003,* http://www.ornl.gov/.

6. Francis Collins and David Galas, "A New Five-Year Plan for the U.S. Human Genome Project," *Science* 262, no. 5130 (1993): 43–46.

7. Office of Management and Budget (OMB), "OMB Directive No. 15: Race and Ethnic Standards for Federal Statistics and Administrative Reporting," adopted May 12, 1977, *Centers for Disease Control and Prevention,* https://wonder.cdc.gov/.

8. Epstein, *Inclusion.*

9. Institute of Medicine, Michael A. Stoto, Ruth Behrens, and Connie Rosemont, eds., *Healthy People 2000: Citizens Chart the Course* (Washington, D.C.: National Academies Press, 1990).

10. "The National Institutes of Health Revitalization Act of 1993," P.L. 103-43, June 10, 1993, *National Institutes of Health,* https://history.nih.gov/research/downloads/pl103-43.pdf.

11. Centers for Disease Control and Prevention, "Use of Race and Ethnicity in Public Health Surveillance: Summary of the CDC/ATSDR Workshop, Atlanta, Georgia, March 1–2, 1993," *MMWR Morbidity and Mortality Weekly Report: Recommendations and Reports* 42, no. RR-10 (1993): 1–16.

12. Reardon, *Race to the Finish.*

13. Ibid.

14. Bliss, *Race Decoded.*

15. UNESCO, "Human Genome Diversity Project," address delivered by Luca Cavalli-Sforza, Stanford University, to a special meeting of UNESCO, September 21, 1994, *SciTech Connect,* http://www.osti.gov/scitech/biblio/505327.

16. Danielle Knight, "Gene Project Deemed Unethical," *Inter Press Service*

News Agency, November 1, 1997, http://www.ipsnews.net/; see also Chee Heng Leng, Laila El-Hamamsy, John Fleming, et al., "Bioethics and Human Population Genetics Research," *UNESCO*, November 15, 1995, http://www.unesco.org/.

17. U.S. Department of Energy, "To Know Ourselves: The U.S. Department of Energy and the Human Genome Project," July 1996, https://archive.org/.

18. Francis S. Collins, Lisa D. Brooks, and Aravinda Chakravarti, "A DNA Polymorphism Discovery Resource for Research on Human Genetic Variation," *Genome Research* 8, no. 12 (1998): 1229–31.

19. Francis S. Collins, Ari Patrinos, Elke Jordan, Aravinda Chakravarti, et al., "New Goals for the U.S. Human Genome Project: 1998–2003," *Science* 282 (1998), 682–83, 688.

20. Rick Weiss, "The Promise of Precision Prescriptions," *Washington Post*, June 24, 2000, https://www.washingtonpost.com/.

21. Derek V. Exner, Daniel L. Dries, Michael J. Domanski, and Jay N. Cohn. "Lesser Response to Angiotensin-Converting-Enzyme Inhibitor Therapy in Black as Compared with White Patients with Left Ventricular Dysfunction," *New England Journal of Medicine* 344, no. 18 (2001): 1351–57; Clyde W. Yancy, Michael B. Fowler, Wilson S. Colucci, et al., "Race and the Response to Adrenergic Blockade with Carvedilol in Patients with Chronic Heart Failure," *New England Journal of Medicine* 344, no. 18 (2001): 1358–65.

22. Robert S. Schwartz, "Racial Profiling in Medical Research," *New England Journal of Medicine* 344 (2001): 1392–93; A. J. Wood, "Racial Differences in the Response to Drugs—Pointers to Genetic Differences," *New England Journal of Medicine* 344 (2001): 1394–96.

23. Alondra Nelson, *Body and Soul: The Black Panther Party and the Fight against Medical Discrimination* (Minneapolis: University of Minnesota Press, 2011).

24. Sheryl Gay Stolberg, "The World: Skin Deep; Shouldn't a Pill Be Colorblind?," *New York Times*, May 13, 2001, http://www.nytimes.com/.

25. Nicholas Wade, "Race Is Seen as Real Guide to Track Roots of Disease," *New York Times*, July 30, 2002, http://www.nytimes.com/.

26. International HapMap Consortium, "The International HapMap Project," *Nature* 426 (2003): 789–96.

27. N. Patil, A. J. Berno, D. A. Hinds, et al., "Blocks of Limited Haplotype Diversity Revealed by High-Resolution Scanning of Human Chromosome 21," *Science* 294 (2001): 1719–23.

28. Catherine Bliss, "Genome Sampling and the Biopolitics of Race," in *A Foucault for the 21st Century: Governmentality Biopolitics and Discipline in the New*, ed. Samuel Binkley and Jorge Capetilla, 322–29 (Newcastle upon Tyne, U.K.: Cambridge Scholars Publishing, 2009).

29. Avram Goldstein and Rick Weiss, "Howard U. Plans Genetics Database," *Washington Post*, May 28, 2003, https://www.washingtonpost.com/.

30. Ibid.

31. Neil Risch, Esteban Burchard, Elad Ziv, and Hua Tang, "Categorization of Humans in Biomedical Research: Genes, Race and Disease," *Genome Biology* 3, no. 7 (2002): comment 2007.

32. Anne L. Taylor, Susan Ziesche, Clyde Yancy, et al., "Combination of Isosorbide Dinitrate and Hydralazine in Blacks with Heart Failure," *New England Journal of Medicine* 351, no. 20 (2004): 2049–57.

33. Jay N. Cohn, "The Use of Race and Ethnicity in Medicine: Lessons from the African-American Heart Failure Trial," *Journal of Law, Medicine, and Ethics* 34, no. 3 (2006): 552–54; Gary Puckrein, "BiDil: From Another Vantage Point," *Health Affairs* 25, no. 5 (2006): w368–74.

34. Jonathan Kahn, "Beyond BiDil: The Expanding Embrace of Race in Biomedical Research and Product Development," *Saint Louis University Journal of Health, Law, and Public Policy* 3 (2009): 61–92.

35. Jonathan Kahn, "Mandating Race: How the USPTO Is Forcing Race into Biotech Patents," *Nature Biotechnology* 29, no. 5 (2011): 401–3.

36. Catherine Bliss, "Translating Racial Genomics: Passages In and Beyond the Lab," *Qualitative Sociology* 36 (2013): 423, and "The Marketization of Identity Politics," *Sociology* 47, no. 5 (2013): 1011–25.

37. Abdullah S. Daar and Peter A. Singer, "Ethics and Geographical Ancestry: Implications for Drug Development and Global Health," *UNESCO* 6, no. 3 (2006): 77; see also Ruha Benjamin, "A Lab of Their Own: Genomic Sovereignty as Postcolonial Policy," *Policy and Society* 28, no. 4 (2009): 341–55; and Ian Whitmarsh, *Biomedical Ambiguity: Race, Asthma, and the Contested Meaning of Genetic Research in the Caribbean* (Ithaca, N.Y.: Cornell University Press, 2008).

38. Anne Fausto-Sterling, "Refashioning Race: DNA and the Politics of Health Care," *Differences* 15, no. 3 (2004): 28.

39. Troy Duster, "Feedback Loops in the Politics of Knowledge Production," in *The Governance of Knowledge*, ed. Nico Stehr, 139–59 (Piscataway, N.J.: Transaction, 2004).

40. "FY 2012 President's Budget for HHS," 2011, and "FY 2013 President's Budget for HHS," 2012, *U.S. Department of Health and Human Services*, http://www.hhs.gov/.

41. "HHS Strategic Plan, Fiscal Years 2007–2012," *U.S. Department of Health and Human Services, Office of the Assistant Secretary for Planning and Evaluation*, September 19, 2007, https://aspe.hhs.gov/.

42. "RFA-CA-09-001: NIH-Supported Centers for Population Health and Health Disparities (CPHHD) (P50)," *National Institutes of Health*, 2009, http://grants.nih.gov/.

43. "Genes, Environment and Health Initiative Invests in Genetic Studies, Environmental Monitoring Technologies," news release, *National Institutes of Health*, September 4, 2007, http://www.nih.gov/.

44. "NIH Health Disparities Strategic Plan, Fiscal Years 2004–2008," *National Human Genome Research Institute*, 2003, https://www.genome.gov/pages/research/der/derreportspublications/nhgrihealthdisparitiesplan.pdf, 12.

45. "Public Health Genomics," *Centers for Disease Control and Prevention*, http://www.cdc.gov/genomics.

46. "NIH Common Fund," *National Institutes of Health*, https://commonfund.nih.gov/.

47. NIH, "Genes, Environment and Health Initiative."

48. GENEVA (Gene Environment Association Studies) study, archived at https://www.genome.gov/27550876/.

49. "NIH Global Health Research Meeting Summary," *National Institutes of Health*, https://commonfund.nih.gov/.

50. Duster, "Selective Arrests."

51. Joan H. Fujimura, Troy Duster, and Ramya Rajagopalan, "Introduction: Race, Genetics, and Disease: Questions of Evidence, Matters of Consequence," in "Race, Genomics, and Biomedicine," edited by Joan H. Fujimura, Troy Duster, and Ramya Rajagopalan, *Social Studies of Science* 38, no. 5 (2008): 643–56.

6
What Do We Owe Each Other?
Moral Debts and Racial Distrust in Experimental Stem Cell Science

RUHA BENJAMIN AND LESLIE R. HINKSON

> The problem of distrusting citizens should be recast or reformulated as an issue of social justice.
> —JOHN M. JOHNSON AND ANDREW MELNIKOV, "WISDOM OF DISTRUST" (2009)

The research design process, the development of therapeutics, and face-to-face clinical encounters—in all of these, biomedicine utilizes ethnoracial categories as salient markers of difference that ostensibly tell us something meaningful about individuals' disease predisposition and health risks. Some proponents of race-based medicine proudly self-identify as racially profiling doctors, arguing that stereotypes are useful because diseases and treatment responses often "cluster by race–ethnicity."[1] Others reluctantly use racial labels as a proxy—one of many indicators that can be utilized in the tool kit of individualized treatment until more precise diagnostics are available. While the literature engaging the more zealous and ambivalent versions of race-based medicine offers many important insights, in the larger public discourse around this issue, the question of what counts as race-based medicine is rarely interrogated.[2] The latter is often presented as a particular set of health interventions rather than as the default setting of medicine in the United States. Whether or not particular racial labels are used, and independent of individual clinicians' intentions or views, the institution of medicine in the United States is characterized by "cultural practices of inequality" that structure health care in ways that are racially disparate.[3]

For example, one study found a significant difference in physicians' nonverbal communication with Black and White patients in end-of-life care. Doctors' exhibited "fewer positive, rapport-building nonverbal cues [e.g., posture, proximity, time spent, and touch] when speaking with black patients."[4] The researchers situate their findings within a broader pattern in which "black patients are more likely than white patients to die in the intensive care unit with life-sustaining treatments," suggesting that differences in doctor communication may contribute to this disparity. Rather than confine analysis to a new drug or technology that explicitly targets patients on the basis of race, we want to highlight how the unequal treatment described above—the subtle but no less deadly variety—should be understood as a more pervasive form of race-based medicine. This more expansive approach to how and when race is meaningful in both medical research and practice is vital to an analysis of the dynamics of trust and trustworthiness. Here we examine the normative underpinnings of "trust talk," asking how biomedical recruitment discourse constructs racial group boundaries within the context of stem cell research (SCR).

In the United States, African Americans have historically been conscripted for experimental medical research while denied access to quality health care.[5] As one informant aptly queried, "Why am I in such demand as a research subject when no one wants me as a patient?" Since the passage of the National Institutes of Health Revitalization Act in 1993, there exists a legal mandate to include a racially diverse population in medical research. This fuels a "vexing and time consuming body hunt" because researchers find it difficult to recruit a representative sample of participants.[6] This purported lack of racial representation is also cause for anxiety in fields that require human tissue samples to hone treatments. In the arena of human SCR, some observers are concerned that the inability of stem cell banks to obtain tissue from a racially diverse population will ultimately make it harder for non-Whites to obtain a tissue match if and when therapies are developed.[7] As one Hastings Center Report contends, "Stem cell therapies should be available to people of all ethnicities. However, most cells used in the clinic will probably come from lines of cells stored in stem cell banks, which may end up benefiting the majority group most."[8] While social scientists and human geneticists have demonstrated how this and similar statements mistakenly conflate racial classifications with genetic diversity, the following analysis raises a different set of issues with respect to such calls for stem cell diversity. A primary reason that researchers and policy analysts provide for the low enrollment of African Americans as clinical subjects or tissue donors is their purported tendency to distrust science and medicine. Hundreds of peer-reviewed articles have been written to discern why, under what circumstances, and with what consequences Africans Americans express distrust.[9] In this way, Black distrust circulates as a biomedical truism, an empirical curiosity, and a cultural trait unique to African Americans—what sociologists of race call an essentialist approach—with little interrogation of the wider discursive field in which it circulates.

In framing trust as a "valued and scarce resource" that some groups purportedly have more of than others, this discussion critically engages the moral economy of cultural and institutional debt and obligation that animates experimental stem cell science.[10] Do African Americans have a moral obligation to their community, and to scientific progress more broadly, to enroll into clinical trials or donate tissue to stem cell banks? Can the medical establishment in general, and experimental medicine in particular, make this claim even as they attempt to redress a history of neglect and often abuse of Black bodies? And can programs designed at least in part to make amends for this past effectively do so without monitoring and questioning the ways in which their current practices are informed by this historical inequality? Trust seems to be the currency through which these moral obligations and historical debts are negotiated. How trust is framed—whether through the lens of group deficit or through examining institutionalized structures of inequality within biomedicine—ultimately determines who is seen as owing as well as what is owed.

By putting the sociology of race/ethnicity in conversation with the social studies of science and medicine, the following analysis extends our understanding of how epistemic and normative practices are inextricable. Well-meaning attempts that use science and medicine to redress prior forms of abuse and neglect are often based on assumptions of inherent racial differences.[11] In particular, Pollock's incisive analysis of Derrida's *pharmakon* metaphor as simultaneously cure and poison best illustrates the tension herein: a race for cures resuscitates static group boundaries in the quest to produce novel medical treatments.[12] However, it is not only biologically reductive notions of race that are revived in stem cell recruitment discourse; culturally essentialist ideas about group traits—trusting versus nontrusting groups—also require critical attention.

In challenging biological determinism, extant scholarship in the social studies of science and medicine has often overlooked the way that reified notions of culture are routinely used as a lens to make sense of group differences.[13] For example, Benjamin found that some clinicians and researchers routinely use generalizations such as "Asian American science-philia" or "African American fatalism" to explain why people choose to participate in experimental stem cell treatments or not.[14] It is worth noting that in these instances, racial logics are typically used in an attempt to include and represent a wider spectrum of the body politic rather than to exclude and dominate, as in previous eras where eugenic ideologies were the norm. The current context is what Epstein has called the inclusion and difference paradigm, whereby "researchers are enjoined to conduct subgroup comparisons by race to test whether treatments have different effects in different groups."[15] In the process, many researchers often mistakenly come to believe that "medical 'have-nots' [are] pounding on the walls of research institutions, demanding to be let into the experimental domain."[16] Yet these same researchers must routinely grapple with resistance or indifference to their solicitations; they often try to make sense of their difficulty in recruiting non-White subjects through the idiom of distrust.[17] By constructing trust as a cultural trait that some groups have more or less of than others, such discursive practices lead those engaged in trust talk to overlook differences within purported ethnoracial groups, to disregard similarities across groups, and most importantly to ignore the larger institutionalized structures of inequality in biomedicine and beyond.

Drawing on a two-year multimethod study of the world's largest stem cell initiative conducted by Benjamin, we interrogate the normative underpinnings of biomedical recruitment discourse.[18] After a discussion of methods and relevant scholarship in this area, we identify three ways in which trust talk in the stem cell field constructs racial group boundaries: through diversity outreach, clinical gatekeeping, and charismatic collaborations. By exploring these practices through three ethnographic vignettes, we also explicate counternarratives—racial profiling, subversive whiteness, and biopolitical minstrelsy—that challenge the normative underpinnings of trust talk in biomedicine. Throughout, we consider how a critical analysis of trust talk in biomedicine relates to broader themes of debt and indebtedness in race-based medicine.

First, part of the push to include more non-White participants in biomedical research—particularly African Americans—is not simply to increase the diversity of research subjects but to do so with the goal of addressing past patterns of race-based neglect. As such, this practice may be interpreted as a form of reparative justice—at least in theory—that attempts to make amends for this history by targeting members of racialized groups in both the recruitment stage and in the treatment and analysis stages of biomedical research. Second, this racial targeting in and of itself contributes to the cultural othering of those this targeting is meant to help. Rather than normalizing their presence and their care over time, such targeting often leads to greater marginalization of African Americans in biomedical research. We illustrate how biomedicine, even and perhaps especially when it proceeds with the intentions of addressing issues of racial reparative justice, is a site of group making, and one that does not simply leave existing social arrangements in place but potentially reifies the racial status quo through a moral economy of trust. By focusing on trust as an exclusively cultural attribute that certain groups innately have more or less of, divorced from sociopolitical context or historical significance, researchers inadvertently frame racial and ethnic groups as either compliant, worthy subjects or less worthy ones whose cultural deficiency undermines scientific progress, hinders attempts to redress past wrongs through greater inclusion, and contributes to their own medical neglect. Thus, those who are owed become those who owe, called on to increase their participation in research as a result of a moral obligation to their racial community and to the greater scientific community. Rather than redress or reparations, then, inclusion turns into a gift of sorts to racialized subjects, one that creates an obligation that can only be met or repaid through some form of bodily sacrifice.

Methods and Background
Inside the Stem Cell Initiative

Stem cells have the potential to regenerate any tissue in the human body—that is, they are pluripotent. However, because many researchers utilize cells taken from the inner lining of a five- to eight-day-old embryo to harness pluripotency, some techniques have proven extremely controversial in the United States. In over a dozen states, initiatives to fund or ban SCR have spurred legislative action or public referendum. Voters approved the single largest funder of SCR in the world, California's Proposition 71, on November 2, 2004. Proposition 71 authorized the sale of general obligation bonds to raise $3 billion over ten years to fund SCR, including contested methods that utilize human embryos to isolate stem cells. The Stem Cell Research and Cures Act in turn amended the state constitution to include a "right to research."[19]

The following discussion draws on findings from Benjamin's two-year (2005–7) mixed-method study of the California Stem Cell Research and Cures Initiative and the California Institute for Regenerative Medicine (CIRM), the new state agency established by Proposition 71. Through a formal affiliation with the agency as part of its first cohort of training fellows, Benjamin observed institute board meetings, scientific retreats, academic courses, legislative and legal hearings, and biotechnology industry conferences; she also conducted content analysis of Proposition 71 campaign finance documents, CIRM press releases, and SCR media documents. Additionally, she interviewed a purposive sample of sixty-three people actively engaged in advocating for, implementing, or critiquing CIRM in the regulatory, biomedical, and civic arenas. This included patients and their families, physicians, and other medical staff who utilized or who provided medical services at an urban teaching hospital, the Garvey Research Complex (a pseudonym). The latter houses a cord blood bank, a stem cell transplant program, and a regional sickle cell clinic, as well as a number of other clinical and research departments.[20]

The fieldwork at Garvey entailed shadowing the head physician in the sickle cell clinic, attending medical rounds, observing patients in clinic visits, and observing discussions between physicians, nurses, and social workers, including discussions on patients' medical and social histories. Benjamin was given access to cord blood program enrollees and observed the process by which parents of children affected by an ailment were instructed to collect and store blood for possible use in a stem cell transplant. Unlike embryonic stem cells, this method for treating sickle cell disease and other blood-based disorders utilizes adult stem cells from a mother's umbilical cord upon giving birth to a child who is not affected by the illness but who might match the affected sibling. Patients and health professionals (including nurses, social workers, outreach workers, doctors, and researchers) were observed in a number of settings, including home visits with patients and their families, sickle cell community events, and community-based talks by scientists working on stem cell transplantation.

In telephone interviews with parents who had banked umbilical cord blood from an unaffected sibling at Garvey's tissue bank for possible future use in a stem cell transfusion, Benjamin asked what factors they were considering as they decided whether and when to have their child undergo transplantation. In examining their attitudes in relation to the broader context of recruitment, Benjamin came to understand that she, as well as those engaged in the new science of recruitment, tended to limit their unit of analysis to individual decision making rather than investigating how institutional norms and discursive practices shape the larger context of meaning making and how these in turn shape racialized views on trust in the biomedical sphere. These findings beg the question of whether reparative schemes can succeed without a full accounting of the cumulative costs associated with past medical wrongs—in this case, how past wrongs create an environment in which trust is not owed to the scientific community for its recent efforts but has yet to be earned.

"Rights" That Do Wrong

The inclusion of racialized groups in research is implicitly framed as a medical right—an extension of biological citizenship—which posits the body as a primary locus of political redress; it is a form of reparative justice, if you will.[21] Scholars have detailed how a history of "deliberate neglect and medical abuse" has led many Black-health advocates to demand biomedical access even as they refuse to participate in experimental research.[22] Thus, a supposed right to access biomedical goods must be understood within a larger sociohistorical context, in which such rights entail the potential to be done wrong and to do wrong. The racialized dimension of rights that can do wrong is particularly acute in the context of experimental stem cell treatments, where researchers seek diverse representation in tissue donation upstream and in clinical trials downstream.

The relationship between advances in the life sciences and new rights that lay claim to those advances is what Jasanoff terms bioconstitutionalism.[23] Through bioconstitutional struggles, legal and social obligations are identified and then become unsettled as the state's political prerogatives are reworked in light of new demands such as diverse stem cell lines. As with affirmative action policies in higher education, a program that was once (arguably) explicitly focused on issues of reparative justice has shifted from addressing the needs of the historically wronged to extolling the benefits of diversity to be realized by the scientific community as a whole through their inclusion. That is, inclusion, previously identified as a tool to further a legal and social obligation of reparative justice, becomes unsettled and is then reworked as a tool for increasing diversity for the sake of the scientific endeavor itself. Most importantly, the issue of what the state owes particular groups is intimately connected to biological definitions of what constitutes a group in the first place. Older forms of group making such as race are not simply replaced by but are often resuscitated in the service of new biopolitical practices that exercise social and political power over the life of racialized subjects, but in ways that either increasingly deny the role of race (color-blindness) or proudly acknowledge its use as a means toward improving the lives of minority subjects (racial profiling). As in other social arenas, individuals' racialized dispositions, and not institutional forms of racism, are typically the locus of concern in popular discourse surrounding trust in biomedicine.[24]

The passage of the California Stem Cell Act can be understood as "a rethinking of law at a constitutional level. At these moments, the most basic relations between states and citizens are reframed through changes in the law."[25] The act was in essence a bioconstitutional moment, where the struggle is over "who we are, what we are owed, and what we are responsible for" as both objects and subjects of scientific initiatives unfolded.[26] In California and a growing number of jurisdictions, representatives of various constituencies attempted to codify answers to these fundamental questions. In the process, histories of medical neglect and scientific abuse, as well as debates over ongoing racial health disparities, were resuscitated and often quickly reburied, lest they slow the urgent race for cures.[27] As a result of this, while biological and cultural notions of race became solidified in answering the question of who, answers concerning what was owed and by whom were obscured and ultimately neglected.

Binaries and Biomedicine

Discursive negotiations are fundamental for the mutual construction of reality, especially as it relates to racial discourse and the construction of Whiteness.[28] The drive to include a diverse population in experimental treatments rests in part on design and recruitment practices informed by a culturally framed binary: White trust versus non-White distrust in biomedicine.[29] This reproduces racial boundaries within a symbolic order in which consent and compliance are implicitly coded White while dissent and refusal are coded non-White. Thus, biomedicine seeks to not only ameliorate bodily suffering but also cultural attitudes toward cure that are rendered pathological. As such, researchers inadvertently extol trust as the desired attitude toward recruitment, even when this conceals the flaws of biomedicine, most notably the vast ethnoracial inequities to which a distrusting attitude may be acutely attuned.

We next identify three ways in which the discourse surrounding trust in the stem cell field constructs racial group boundaries: diversity outreach, clinical gatekeeping, and charismatic collaborations. We also explicate corresponding counternarratives, including medical racial profiling, subversive whiteness, and biopolitical minstrelsy, as forms of discursive resistance that challenge standard recruitment norms. In examining these, we hope to shed light on the limitations of current biomedical rhetoric and practice to engage the concerns of socially subordinated groups, and ultimately to reorient the moral economy of trust in biomedical research.

Recruitment and Its Discontents
Diversity Outreach and Racial Profiling

On October 14, 2006, a group of scientists, clinicians, social justice advocates, health policy analysts, and academics participated in a conference in Oakland, California, entitled "Toward Fair Cures: Integrating the Benefits of Diversity in the California Stem Cell Research Act," sponsored by the UC Berkeley Project on Stem Cells and Society, the Children's Hospital of Oakland Research Institute, and the Greenlining Institute (a national policy, grassroots organizing, and leadership training institute working for racial and economic justice). The purpose of the event was to "increase the understanding of the economic and medical potential of stem cell research among historically underserved minority communities and ensure that California's stem cell research efforts serve our state's diverse community."[30] A point of debate was the conference's subtitle: "Addressing the *Lack* of Diversity in Stem Cell Research." Organizers were forced to change this to the more upbeat title, "Integrating the *Benefits* of Diversity in the California Stem Cell Research Act" (italics added) when cosponsor Robert Birgeneau, UC Berkeley's chancellor, told them it was too confrontational.[31] However, key organizers maintained that this reframing undermined the autonomy and agency of health policy advocates to address the historic exclusion and exploitation of racialized groups in scientific and medical decision making.

Birgeneau's intervention highlights a larger pattern that sociologists Bell and Hartman describe as the ubiquity of diversity "happy talk" in U.S. discourse on race and ethnicity—a way of addressing race that is sanitized as a result of the "cultural blind spots" that reinforce White normativity and fail to consider the effects of the "unseen privileges and normative presumptions" of mainstream American culture.[32] Attempting to unsettle this normative center, several conference participants underscored the fact that if tax-spending decisions were made in an inclusive way and reflected the values, interests, and perspectives of truly diverse groups, SCR would not top the list. One conference participant observed that "all technology has power relations embedded in [it], [is] developed to benefit specific populations and [is] made available to specific populations. [. . .] If we were to go to minority communities and women's communities and ask them how to spend $3 to $6 billion, it's unlikely that they would say 'on stem cell research.'"[33] Given that a significant portion of racialized individuals face obstacles to accessing even the most basic medical care, this statement rings true.

Similarly, another participant urged attendees to shift the focus away from minority distrust in science to the "trustworthiness of institutions."[34] While this provocation was not taken up as a major locus of concern for participants, it serves as a window into the way that discourses around trust in biomedicine typically pivot around the disposition of individuals and groups rather than focus on the norms and practices associated with institutions. From the latter perspective, what is often called outreach relies on group profiling, where the discourse surrounding trust is a major feature of constructing ethnoracial profiles.

Consider, for example, a diversity workshop at the Charles R. Drew University of Medicine and Science, hosted by the state stem cell agency on February 26, 2010. Drew is a historically Black institution founded in Los Angeles' Watts neighborhood in response to the 1965 urban rebellion sparked by social and economic oppression that Blacks faced and continue to face. Its mission today is to educate and serve the predominantly Black and Hispanic residents of the area. The goals of the diversity workshop were twofold: to "gain a greater understanding of how population diversity affects, benefits and advances CIRM's mission" and "to use this knowledge to ensure that CIRM's funding initiatives support diversity in regenerative medicine." During this workshop, an invited speaker, Dr. Maria Pallavicini, explained how the University of California, Merced, had to "educate the population of this historically underserved population in the San Joaquin Valley about the nature and value of research." This, she said, had been "a challenge in a region with relatively high rates of poverty and low levels of educational achievement."[35]

Another speaker, Dr. Keith Norris of Drew University, highlighted the importance of research scientists engaging with doctors and clinical researchers, and underscored that the goal of this interaction "should be to relate research to broader community health concerns."[36] Reflecting a deficit framing of patient compliance and participation (i.e., focused on what people lack), Norris observed that "functional illiteracy" ("48 percent of U.S. adults cannot fill out a job application") limits people's ability to participate in research initiatives. He also mentioned other socioeconomic factors, such as "concerns about the time and expenses (travel, child care, lost income)," that hinder participation in research studies. Accordingly, Norris suggested that "smaller mission-based and/or minority-serving institutions," like Drew University, could be a potential resource for increasing minority participation in research. Norris did not speculate on the possible deficiencies of the institution of medical research in its ability to recruit more broadly, and he made no mention of how the research enterprise itself may have contributed to lower levels of patient compliance and participation.

Relatedly, scientists at the CIRM diversity workshop emphasized the importance of developing a "diverse stock of cells" to ensure immune tolerability across the diverse population who will seek access to future cell-based therapies. Dr. Louise Laurent of UC San Diego presented "results from genetic analysis indicating there is restricted genetic diversity in established human embryonic stem cell lines." In other words, because many stem cell lines are produced using eggs from fertility clinics whose donors are predominantly non-Hispanic whites, the stem cell lines disproportionately catered to that demographic. The UC San Diego team stressed that it was "developing a genetically diverse collection of human iPS cell lines.... The success of this effort depends, in part, on the ability to recruit a genetically diverse group of donors to participate in the project."[37] Laurent's concerns drew on prior "considerations of justice in stem cell research and therapy" that warned that a lack of ethnoracial diversity would necessarily result in a lack of genetic diversity and the subsequent exclusion of groups who were not well represented in basic research and tissue biobanks.[38] Reiterating the findings from the Hastings report, "Unless the problem of biological access is carefully addressed, an American stem cell bank may end up benefiting primarily white Americans, to the relative exclusion of the rest of the population."[39] Again, genetic diversity is conflated with reified U.S. racial categories. From this perspective, while existing levels of diversity in these stem cell banks seem adequate to address the genetic diversity that truly describes White America, they are not diverse enough to serve the needs of the nation's racial others.

Conference-goers in turn relied on cultural explanations for non-Whites' lack of participation. One CIRM study presentation, "Supporting Diversity in Research Participation: A Framework for Action," attributed nonparticipation to people of color's lack of understanding about clinical trials and their risks and benefits, literacy deficits, and finally "a general lack of trust in the health care system and especially in clinical research."

> African-Americans tend to have the lowest level of trust in the health care system because of historical abuses. Chinese-Americans also have

trust issues, as well as problems with English and . . . older members of the community and recent immigrants [have] a lack of understanding of the underlying concepts of clinical research. Latinos also face language barriers, as well as a fear on the part of immigrants—legal or otherwise—that participation could bring negative consequences for them and their families [i.e., deportation]. Southeast Asians share many of these issues, along with, for many groups, a fear of authority bred by a variety of traumas.[40]

In short, while the White versus non-White boundary is implicitly reinforced by describing the aforementioned groups as all having trust issues, they are given distinct profiles in which history, language, and education among other factors are used to make sense of their ambivalence toward biomedical recruitment. Accordingly, these profiles are recommended for use by researchers attempting to successfully recruit non-Whites for inclusion in their trials. Thus, as in quests for diversity more broadly, inclusion rests upon reified notions of difference that often leave institutional structures unexamined.

Embedded in the hard-to-reach framing of minority recruitment was the idea that their relative proximity to biomedicine was a matter of self-selection rather than systemic dispossession. While references to African Americans' historic distrust—particularly the oft-mentioned Tuskegee Syphilis Study (1932–72)—suggested external justification for why some people might be hard to reach, issues of ongoing social marginality were largely absent from conference conversations. In particular, social production of distrust in racialized groups via daily encounters with the U.S. health care system and lack of access were not mentioned.[41] But whereas diversity outreach discourse obscures such inequities, the unhappy talk of medical racial profiling alerts us to the normative underpinnings of recruitment efforts. If increasing recruitment of subordinated racial groups is a necessary condition for addressing past biomedical wrongs and repaying its past debts, then these normative underpinnings must be critically examined and countered as a first step toward building more trustworthy institutions.

Clinical Gatekeepers and Subversive Whiteness

At Garvey Research Complex, a related dynamic ensued as primary care physicians—the "crucial mediators between patients and clinical researchers"—formed an intermediary tier of distrust that is all but invisible in the larger discourse of biomedical recruitment.[42] Namely, some

White clinicians are at odds with researchers, surgeons, and specialists over the efficacy of new high-tech treatments and expensive drugs. Therefore, they exhibit their own brand of ambivalence and distrust; they can be described as subversive within the larger context of what sociologist Matthew Hughey calls hegemonic whiteness, a term Hughey uses to capture the fact that "while there is no question about the political differences and individual heterogeneity of white actors in an array of settings, it is important to recognize that certain forms of whiteness can become dominant and pursued as an ideal."[43] In this case, the idealization of trusting patients and compliant research subjects, implicitly coded White, is reinforced when recruitment discourse fails to adequately account for the ways that clinicians themselves may subvert the dominant narrative about medical institutions as altruistic and trustworthy.

Take, for example, Garvey physician Tate Wright, who regularly attributes patient noncompliance to the stress of his patients' daily lives and the ineffectiveness of prescribed treatments. As a member of a predominantly White clinical staff serving a Black patient population, he was acutely aware of racial and power asymmetries and how these could inhibit patient trust and compliance. He disagreed with other hospitals' behavior contracts, which are often selectively applied to young Black patients, particularly the zero-tolerance policies that are maintained: "Failure to comply with the following rules will result in your immediate discharge from the hospital and/or the intervention of law enforcement personnel."[44]

One afternoon, in the sickle cell anemia clinic, he shared a story of fifteen-year-old Tyrone Hemmingway. Tyrone and his family had elected to remove his spleen, because, as is common with sickle cell anemia, it became swollen as the sickled hemoglobin blocked the blood vessels. Wright explained:

> The doctor who performed the surgery decided to use some high-tech equipment that would allow him to do a laser surgery, which meant that he wouldn't have to open Tyrone all the way up. But because Tyrone's spleen was so big and they couldn't finish the operation in a reasonable amount of time, they left him open, iced his stomach and wrapped him up. They brought him back to complete the surgery the following day, because they didn't want to keep him under anesthetics so long in his condition. But in the second round they accidentally lacerated his stomach, although they didn't yet know it. So they sewed him up and when he got back into his room, he was complaining of pain. Staff thought it was just the post-op pain. Then he started peeing

black urine and vomiting up blood. So they rushed him back into the operating room and opened him up and found the tear in his stomach. A few days later, Tyrone was still saying he was in a lot of pain, and it turned out that although they sewed the tear, he was digesting his pancreas.[45]

Wright recounted the half dozen surgeries in three weeks that were required to rectify the initial surgical damage. When he visited Tyrone after one of these surgeries, he "honestly didn't think this kid was going to make it." Wright further mused, "The family has been *so good* about it. I mean they are angry, but they're not enraged like they *ought* to be. I mean it was an elective surgery, and the poor mom, every time she left the hospital they called her to say that Tyrone was being rushed into the emergency room."[46]

In a related fashion, Wright expressed his ambivalence toward the newest technique on the block alongside his disdain for his colleagues' career-advancing motivations. In one instance, in the midst of explaining that a new hemoglobin had been discovered at the Garvey Research Complex, he stated that the institution "is a little tacky since you're supposed to name it after the patient, *not* the person who discovers it." When a new medical student asked a round of questions about the discovery process, he said, "A lot of what's driving the discovery of hemoglobin types is scientists trying to get their report in *Blood* [a medical journal], even if it's just based on one patient and the type is never seen again." Finally, Wright and others at Garvey avoided referring patients to other specialists whose decisions they questioned and who were supportive of experimental procedures like the stem cell transplantation that was then being offered in the research wing of the hospital. In all these ways, Wright exemplified what we are calling subversive Whiteness insofar as he used his position as clinical gatekeeper to question and circumvent the recruitment norms of biomedicine. As previously mentioned, his subversion can be understood in the context of what Hughey describes as hegemonic whiteness—an ideal that Tate Wright was deliberately compromising.

As Wailoo and Pemberton document in *The Troubled Dream of Genetic Medicine,* the expectations of those affected by sickle cell disease have repeatedly been raised by pronouncements of breakthrough cures such that, unlike other ailments for which stem cell cures are predicted, there exists an extremely ambivalent relationship between those affected by sickle cell disease and cutting-edge, high-risk medical research.[47] Physicians like Wright are appalled at the "rollercoaster of unfulfilled therapeutic promises."[48] Positioning themselves as allies to their patients, doctors like

Wright act as refusers of the allure of experimental treatments.[49] Still, the cultural conception of distrust as inherently pathological, indicative of a lack of health literacy, and seemingly innate to non-Whites fails to account for Wright's disdain for biomedical business as usual.

Whiteness—not only in terms of Wright's ethnoracial identity but even more so as it is exercised through the authority assigned to the white coat of medicine and science—allows for his distrust to go unmarked, thereby bolstering the binary opposition between non-White distrust and White trust. By focusing only on his role as gatekeeper, we may overlook the way in which he and other clinicians exercise forms of subversion that run counter to the recruitment norms of the stem cell field and other experimental life sciences. This myopia also overlooks how these subversive practices can be harnessed to hold the medical establishment responsible for debts owed to non-White patients—both past and present—as well as to develop relationships of trust between non-White patients and those clinical actors who deserve their trust.

Charismatic Collaborations and Biopolitical Minstrelsy

The final vignette of biomedical recruitment and its relationship to both trust discourse and debt examines charismatic research enthusiasts and the way that their advocacy resists the reification of group boundaries while simultaneously obscuring the power relations that characterize the recruitment process. Richard Gaskin, an African American stem cell activist who was paralyzed from a gunshot wound when he was twenty years old, publicly enacts trust, thus delinking the discursive association of Blackness with distrust. Gaskin's rap moniker, Professir X, draws on the X-Men comic book series about mutant characters with physical characteristics that can be viewed as liabilities or powers. As with the fictional leader of mutants who trains those with seeming disabilities to transform these disabilities into a resource, Gaskin set out to purposefully intervene in the stem cell battles as someone who appears to fully support the new field. Since his injury, he has worked with Michael J. Fox, the late senator Ted Kennedy, and the late Dana Reeve (wife of the late Christopher Reeve) to generate awareness and funds for SCR.[50]

In a 2007 interview, Gaskin expressed the belief that his experience was representative of broader Black sentiment: "Before, there was nobody famous who represented me, except maybe Teddy Pendergrass. . . . Here was somebody who was going out there, fighting for a cure, advocating for better quality of life for people with disabilities, something I'd seen no one else do."[51] After Christopher Reeve's death, Gaskin wrote a song entitled "Forever Superman" about his fellow enthusiast's search for a cure. His song inspired Dr. Wise Young, founder of the W. M. Keck Center for Collaborative Neuroscience, to recruit Gaskin to "[bring] a hip-hop vibe to the world of [spinal cord injury] education and advocacy."[52] Gaskin also traveled to China as a SCR ambassador, thereby aiding Young and the CIRM establishment in framing participation in terms of access to SCR[53]:

> The cost of holding clinical trials—which includes admitting 240 people [the typical size of a phase 1 [clinical] trial into the hospital, tests and treatments, and months of physical therapy—will be about $32 million. So Young and others came up with the JustaDollarPlease.org campaign, asking families and friends of spinal cord injured [people] to give a dollar a day ($365 a year) and everyone to give whatever they can.[54]

Gaskin also elaborates the day-to-day struggle of living with a disability in order to stand in for what he considers the community of patients in need.

The practice of speaking for others is not without its hazards because, as sociologist of science Michel Callon puts it, "to speak for others is to first silence those in whose name we speak."[55] As such, spokespersons like Gaskin do not simply represent; they also help produce a normative ideal of trusting patients in waiting. Charismatic enthusiasts combine rhetoric and reality with the symbolic and the material world, effectively prioritizing the pragmatic requirements of basic research over Black recruitment concerns. For example, sociologist Steven Epstein recounts how one young African American physician was "invited to be a co-investigator on a study, only to conclude eventually that what the senior investigator really sought was a 'black face' to display at community forums for purposes of reassuring potential participants."[56] Indeed, Yancey and colleagues point out, "A common approach to building trust and alleviating attitudinal barriers was community involvement, particularly in the form of using lay outreach workers from the targeted population. Inclusion of minority ('cultural insider') investigators was also advanced as a community engagement strategy . . . [as was the use of] churches [that] provide captive audiences."[57] The use of in-group members as fronts and spokespersons for research initiatives emerges as a way to mitigate distrust and appear more culturally competent. While superficial approaches like this abound, we nevertheless find examples of stem cell recruitment that attempt to transform "the power imbalance between the researcher and the community under study" by involving community spokespeople at earlier stages of the research process to provide input into research questions and protocol.[58] However, in such cases, we are still confronted with difficulties plaguing other efforts at participatory science, many of which are tied to the politics of representation. After all, scientific knowledge "does not simply represent (in the sense of *depict*) 'nature,' but it also represents (in the *political sense*) the 'social interests' of the people and institutions that have become wrapped up in its production."[59]

To some extent, then, charismatic collaborations between researchers and community spokesmen are forged mainly to celebrate and bolster science. However, without building in critical assessments of the impact and meaning of a given field on those targeted as prospective research subjects or tissue donors, public displays of Black trust may enact a kind of biopolitical minstrelsy. Historical analyses of minstrelsy's audiences emphasize the "contradictory impulses at work" rather than conceiving such performances as "uncomplicated or monolithic"; so too does our use of the term signal the unsettled discursive terrain of charismatic collaborations. As Lott describes, "The minstrel show was less the incarnation of an age-old racism than an emergent social semantic figure highly responsive to the emotional demands and troubled fantasies of its audiences . . . [a] mixed erotic economy of celebration and exploitation, what Homi Bhabha would call its 'ambivalence.'"[60] So by biopolitical minstrelsy, we mean the borrowing of Black cultural materials (in this case, hip-hop aesthetics) in the service of powerful scientific and medical institutions to take control over and administer life—a borrowing that serves to obscure the power relations between researchers and African American communities. Ironically, it is this power imbalance that makes such performances necessary in the first place.[61] Thus, biopolitical minstrelsy attempts to elicit behavior in the form of trust from a population that is keenly aware of the imbalanced power dynamics and attuned to historical forces that would deem such trust to be unfounded, as such behavior signals at most a forgiveness of past wrongs and at the least a forgiveness of past debts.

Like Tate Wright, whose own complex role within Garvey elides easy representation in the binary framework of Black distrust and White trust, so too does Professir X's exuberant commitment to the stem cell cause challenge the epistemological bedrock of biomedical recruitment. These seeming exceptions to the discursive linkage between race and trust, and the fact that they stand out as such, serve to underscore both the power and limits of the assumptions that are often made about group dispositions toward experimental biomedicine. They also illustrate that in any attempt to right the wrongs perpetuated by the biomedical establishment in the past, what may be owed is not simply inclusion of previously neglected populations in clinical trials or access to cutting-edge technology. Earnest attempts must be made to own up to past abuses and current discriminatory practices to earn the trust of racially subordinated groups in order to give such reparative schemes any chance of success.

Conclusion

The cultural concept of trust is racialized in the context of biomedicine. We find a binary opposition between White trust and non-White distrust, which structures the moral economy of debt and obligation in the context of experimental biomedicine. Thus, not only do science and medicine tend to affect racially defined groups differently, but also racial logics help to define the norms and practices of science and medicine—a feedback loop that deserves critical attention. Drawing on Cheryl Harris's classic essay "Whiteness as Property," Reardon and TallBear explain that "we live in times where for many, the relevant 'civilizing' project that shapes their lives is the development of the 'knowledge society' in which knowledge is a primary source of wealth."[62] Ideas about ethnoracial groups that assume they are characterized by inherent biological or cultural differences, even in order to ultimately help oppressed communities or to repay historical debts, are an extension of this civilizing logic. As an idea "that brings good things to all, whiteness itself becomes a thing of value that should be developed and defended."[63] Resistance to and distrust of biomedical recruitment in turn becomes a problematic attitude to be cured in the name of scientific progress.

Buying into the value of research is not only or primarily about a philosophical commitment to defending the civilizing mission of biomedicine. It is also a matter of practicality—that is, having the resources to spend on this increasingly costly embrace of biomedicine. As Good declares, "While the world's dominant economies invest private and public monies in the production of biotechnology and aggressively seek to integrate these advances into clinical practice—thereby reaping financial as well as scientific returns on [often tax-funded] capital investments—all societies are confronted with difficult questions about rationing biomedical interventions assumed central to competent clinical medicine."[64] Considering the reality that access to quality health care in the United States is indeed rationed—often along class and racial lines—an attitude of distrust casts a shadow over the logic of research subject recruitment. Does it make sense for non-Whites to participate in clinical trials that may indeed offer medical benefits to their demographic in theory, while inequitable access to quality care makes it impossible for many poor and non-White people to reap those benefits in reality? Whiteness is not simply tied to White bodies or an imagined White culture. It is a larger expression of a calculating modern rationality, which gave rise to *Homo economicus*, that "anthropological monster" whom we might imagine as objectively weighing the risks and benefits of a particular recruitment pitch.[65] Yet when this abstraction is faced with a reality in which research participants may not be able to access the fruits of SCR and other novel treatments, the possible wisdom of distrust becomes apparent. If the biomedical community is serious about repaying past debts to communities it has previously wronged, inclusion should not begin and end with the recruitment process. Instead, it needs to extend throughout the whole biomedical apparatus. Without access to the care and cures their participation in clinical trials and tissue donations promise, members of racially subordinated groups will have few reasons to expect that the exploitative nature of biomedicine is truly a thing of the past.

Notes

Research for this article was made possible through funding and support from the National Science Foundation, the California Institute for Regenerative Medicine, and University of California–Los Angeles' Institute for Society and Genetics. Sincere thanks to the many fieldwork informants who shared their experiences, anonymous peer reviewers, and volume editors who steered this chapter to completion.

1. See Sally Satel, "I Am a Racially Profiling Doctor," *New York Times Magazine*, March 5, 2002, http://www.nytimes.com/.

2. Steven Epstein, *Inclusion: The Politics of Difference in Medical Research* (Chicago: University of Chicago Press, 2007); Jonathan Kahn, *Race in a Bottle: The Story of BiDil and Racialized Medicine* (New York: Columbia University Press, 2012); Dorothy Roberts, *Fatal Invention: How Science, Politics, and Big Business Recreate Race in the Twenty-First Century* (New York: The New Press, 2011).

3. Imani Perry. *More Beautiful and More Terrible: The Embrace and Transcendence of Racial Inequality in the United States* (New York: New York University Press, 2011).

4. Andrea M. Elliott, Stewart C. Alexander, Craig A. Mescher, Deepika Mohan, and Amber E. Barnato, "Differences in Physicians' Verbal and Nonverbal Communication with Black and White Patients at the End of Life," *Journal of Pain and Symptom Management* 51, no. 1 (2016): 1–8.

5. Giselle Corbie-Smith, Stephen B. Thomas, Mark V. Williams, and Sandra

MoodyAyers, "Attitudes and Beliefs of African Americans toward Participation in Medical Research," *Journal of General Internal Medicine* 14, no. 9 (1999): 537–46; Alondra Nelson, *Body and Soul: The Black Panther Party and the Fight against Medical Discrimination* (Minneapolis: University of Minnesota Press, 2011); Keith Wailoo, *Dying in the City of the Blues: Sickle Cell Anemia and the Politics of Race and Health* (Chapel Hill: University of North Carolina Press, 2006); Harriet A. Washington, *Medical Apartheid: The Dark History of Medical Experimentation on Black Americans from Colonial Times to the Present* (New York: Doubleday, 2007). The best-known illustration of the tension between biomedical research and health care is the Tuskegee Syphilis Study, which "became a symbol of their mistreatment by the medical establishment, a metaphor for deceit, conspiracy, malpractice, and neglect, if not outright racial genocide." Corbie-Smith et al., "Attitudes and Beliefs" 542.

6. Steven Epstein, "The Rise of 'Recruitmentology': Clinical Research, Racial Knowledge, and the Politics of Inclusion and Difference," *Social Studies of Science* 38, no. 5 (2008): 806.

7. Ruth R. Faden, Liza Dawson, Alison S. Bateman-House, et al., "Public Stem Cell Banks: Considerations of Justice in Stem Cell Research and Therapy," *Hastings Center Report* 33, no. 6 (2003): 13–27.

8. Mark Greene, "To Restore FAITH and TRUST: Justice and Biological Access to Cellular Therapies," *Hastings Center Report* 36, no. 1 (2006): 57.

9. A comprehensive review of recruitment studies found that for African Americans especially, "perceptions of trust and mistrust of scientific investigators, of government, and of academic institutions were found to be a central barrier to recruitment." Antoinette K. Yancey, Alexander N. Ortega, and Shiriki K. Kumanyika, "Effective Recruitment and Retention of Minority Research Participants," *Annual Review of Public Health* 27 (2006): 9. Research reported that recruitment techniques targeting African Americans (including mass mailings, media campaigns, physician referrals, support groups, health fairs, and community outreach in churches, beauty shops, and barbershops) typically focus on the discrete attitudes of individuals as they work to extend the right of participation to a racially/ethnically representative sample of the U.S. population. See Joel B. Braunstein, Noelle S. Sherber, Steven P. Schulman, Eric L. Ding, and Neil R. Powe, "Race, Medical Researcher Distrust, Perceived Harm, and Willingness to Participate in Cardiovascular Prevention Trials," *Medicine* 87, no. 1 (2008): 1–9; Corbie-Smith et al., "Attitudes and Beliefs"; Annette Dula, "African American Suspicion of the Healthcare System Is Justified: What Do We Do About It?," *Cambridge Quarterly of Healthcare Ethics* 3, no. 03 (1994): 347–57; Vanessa Northington Gamble, "Under the Shadow of Tuskegee: African Americans and Health Care," *American Journal of Public Health* 87, no. 11 (1997): 1773–78; Philip B. Gorelick, Yvonne Harris, Barbara Burnett, and Faith J. Bonecutter, "The Recruitment Triangle: Rea-

sons Why African Americans Enroll, Refuse to Enroll, or Voluntarily Withdraw from a Clinical Trial. An Interim Report from the African-American Antiplatelet Stroke Prevention Study (AAASPS)," *Journal of the National Medical Association* 90, no. 3 (1998): 141; Yvonne Harris, Philip B. Gorelick, Patricia Samuels, and Isaac Bempong, "Why African Americans May Not Be Participating in Clinical Trials," *Journal of the National Medical Association* 88, no. 10 (1996): 630; Vernellia R. Randall, "Slavery, Segregation and Racism: Trusting the Health Care System Ain't Always Easy—An African American Perspective on Bioethics," *St. Louis University Public Law Review* 15 (1995): 191; Charmaine Royal, Agnes Baffoe-Bonnie, Rick Kittles, et al., "Recruitment Experience in the First Phase of the African American Hereditary Prostate Cancer (AAHPC) Study," *Annals of Epidemiology* 10, no. 8 (2000): S68–77.

10. Barbara Misztal. *Trust in Modern Societies: The Search for the Bases of Social Order* (Hoboken, N.J.: Wiley, 2013).

11. Catherine Bliss, *Race Decoded: The Genomic Fight for Social Justice* (Stanford, Calif.: Stanford University Press, 2012); Lundy Braun, Anne Fausto-Sterling, Duana Fullwiley, et al., "Racial Categories in Medical Practice: How Useful Are They?," *PLoS Medicine* 4, no. 9 (2007): e271; Duana Fullwiley, "The Biologistical Construction of Race: 'Admixture' Technology and the New Genetic Medicine," *Social Studies of Science* 38, no. 5 (2008): 695–735; Joan H. Fujimura, Troy Duster, and Ramya Rajagopalan, "Introduction: Race, Genetics, and Disease: Questions of Evidence, Matters of Consequence," in "Race, Genomics, and Biomedicine," edited by Joan H. Fujimura, Troy Duster, and Ramya Rajagopalan, *Social Studies of Science* 38, no. 5 (2008): 643–56; Sandra Soo-Jin Lee, "Racializing Drug Design: Implications of Pharmacogenomics for Health Disparities," *American Journal of Public Health* 95, no. 12 (2005): 2133–38; Michael Montoya, *Making the Mexican Diabetic: Race, Science, and the Genetics of Inequality* (Berkeley: University of California Press, 2011); Pilar Ossorio and Troy Duster, "Race and Genetics: Controversies in Biomedical, Behavioral, and Forensic Sciences," *American Psychologist* 60, no. 1 (2005): 115; Jenny Reardon, *Race to the Finish: Identity and Governance in an Age of Genomics* (Princeton, N.J.: Princeton University Press, 2004).

12. Anne Pollock, *Medicating Race: Heart Disease and Durable Preoccupations with Difference* (Durham, N.C.: Duke University Press, 2012). The notion that society (in the form of reified conceptions of race) and biology (in the form of stem cells that can regenerative human tissue) are coproduced is central to the field of science and technology studies. See Reardon, *Race to the Finish*; Sheila Jasanoff, *Designs on Nature: Science and Democracy in Europe and the United States* (Princeton, N.J.: Princeton University Press, 2005); and Charis Thompson, *Making Parents: The Ontological Choreography of Reproductive Technologies* (Cambridge, Mass.: MIT Press, 2005).

13. For notable exceptions, see Angela C. Jenks, "What's the Use of Culture? Health Disparities and the Development of Culturally Competent Health Care," in *What's the Use of Race? Modern Governance and the Biology of Difference*, ed. David S. Jones and Ian Whitmarsh (Cambridge, Mass.: MIT Press, 2010), 207–24; and Janet K. Shim, "Cultural Health Capital: A Theoretical Approach to Understanding Health Care Interactions and the Dynamics of Unequal Treatment," *Journal of Health and Social Behavior* 51, no. 1 (2010): 1–15.

14. Ruha Benjamin. *People's Science: Bodies and Rights on the Stem Cell Frontier* (Stanford, Calif.: Stanford University Press, 2013).

15. Epstein, "Rise of 'Recruitmentology,'" 813.

16. Ibid., 806.

17. Sociologist of science Charis Thompson, in *Making Parents*, aptly and succinctly describes trust as "what must be unquestioned for any system of truth to be sustained" (41).

18. Benjamin, *People's Science*.

19. Mark B. Brown and David H. Guston, "Science, Democracy, and the Right to Research," *Science and Engineering Ethics* 15, no. 3 (2009): 351–66; Chris Ganchoff, "Regenerating Movements: Embryonic Stem Cells and the Politics of Potentiality," *Sociology of Health and Illness* 26, no. 6 (2004): 757–74.

20. Institutional Review Board human subjects approval #2007-007.

21. Adriana Petryna, *Life Exposed: Biological Citizens after Chernobyl* (Princeton, N.J.: Princeton University Press, 2013); Nikolas Rose and Carlos Novas, "Biological Citizenship," in *Global Assemblages: Technology, Politics, and Ethics as Anthropological Problems,* ed. Aihwa Ong and Stephen Collier, 439–63. (Oxford: Wiley-Blackwell, 2004); Roberts, *Fatal Invention*.

22. Nelson, *Body and Soul*, 15.

23. Sheila Jasanoff, *Reframing Rights: Bioconstitutionalism in the Genetic Age* (Cambridge, Mass.: MIT Press, 2011).

24. Eduardo Bonilla-Silva, *Racism without Racists: Color-blind Racism and the Persistence of Racial Inequality in the United States* (Lanham, Md.: Rowman & Littlefield, 2006).

25. Jasanoff, *Reframing Rights*, 3.

26. Benjamin, *People's Science*, 3.

27. Ossorio and Duster, "Race and Genetics."

28. On construction of reality, see Peter L. Berger and Thomas Luckmann, *The Social Construction of Reality: A Treatise in the Sociology of Knowledge* (New York: Anchor Books, 1967); Erving Goffman, *Interaction Ritual: Essays on Face-to-Face Interaction* (New York: Anchor Books, 1967); C. Wright Mills, "Situated Actions and Vocabularies of Motive," *American Sociological Review* 5, no. 6 (1940): 904–13. On racial discourse, see Simon Goodman and Shani Burke, "'Oh You Don't Want Asylum Seekers, Oh You're Just Racist': A Discursive Analysis of Discussions about Whether It's Racist to Oppose Asylum Seeking," *Discourse*

and Society 21, no. 3 (2010): 325–40; Kristen A. Myers, *Racetalk: Racism Hiding in Plain Sight* (Lanham, Md.: Rowman & Littlefield, 2005); Kristen A. Myers and Passion Williamson, "Race Talk: The Perpetuation of Racism through Private Discourse," *Race and Society* 4, no. 1 (2001): 3–26; Mica Pollock, *Colormute: Race Talk Dilemmas in an American School* (Princeton, N.J.: Princeton University Press, 2009); Martin Reisigl and Ruth Wodak, *Discourse and Discrimination: Rhetorics of Racism and Antisemitism* (London: Routledge, 2001); Margaret Wetherell and Jonathan Potter, *Mapping the Language of Racism: Discourse and the Legitimation of Exploitation* (New York: Columbia University Press, 1992). On the construction of whiteness, see John D. Foster, "Defending Whiteness Indirectly: A Synthetic Approach to Race Discourse Analysis," *Discourse and Society* 20, no. 6 (2009): 685–703; Matthew W. Hughey, "Backstage Discourse and the Reproduction of White Masculinities," *Sociological Quarterly* 52, no. 1 (2011): 132–53; Matthew W. Hughey, *White Bound: Nationalists, Antiracists, and the Shared Meanings of Race* (Stanford, Calif.: Stanford University Press, 2012); Leslie Houts Picca and Joe R. Feagin, *Two-Faced Racism: Whites in the Backstage and Frontstage* (New York: Routledge, 2007); Damien W. Riggs and Martha Augoustinos, "Projecting Threat: Managing Subjective Investments in Whiteness," *Psychoanalysis, Culture, and Society* 9, no. 2 (2004): 219–36; Melissa Steyn and Don Foster, "Repertoires for Talking White: Resistant Whiteness in Post-apartheid South Africa," *Ethnic and Racial Studies* 31, no. 1 (2008): 25–51.

29. Analysts have long established trust "as a critical aspect of medical care . . . that includes perceptions of the health care provider's technical ability, interpersonal skills, and the extent to which the patient perceives that his or her welfare is placed above other considerations." Chanita Hughes Halbert, Katrina Armstrong, Oscar H. Gandy, and Lee Shaker, "Racial Differences in Trust in Health Care Providers," *Archives of Internal Medicine* 166, no. 8 (2006): 896. For example, Epstein emphasizes the "highly charged politics of trust and mistrust that characterize relations between researchers and many communities from which they hope to recruit" ("Rise of 'Recruitmentology,'" 803). Recent studies have gone on to distinguish between interpersonal and societal distrust, where interpersonal distrust is "based on personal experiences and interactions of individuals within health care or clinical research settings" and societal distrust is "characterized by a global negative outlook on clinical research based on perceptions of collective research entities or life experiences in society at large." Reagan W. Durant, Anna T. Legedza, Edward R. Marcantonio, Marcie B. Freeman, and Bruce E. Landon, "Different Types of Distrust in Clinical Research Among Whites and African Americans," *Journal of the National Medical Association* 103, no. 2 (2011): 123, 124. While there are no significant racial differences in interpersonal distrust in clinical research, African Americans are shown to express more societal distrust in clinical research than Whites. So even if individuals trust their doctor, they may refuse to participate in clinical trials and other

forms of experimental treatment because of their experiences with the medical establishment and other social institutions.

30. From the Toward Fair Cures conference publicity material.

31. Personal interview with Joseph Tayag, November 18, 2006, Berkeley, California.

32. Joyce M. Bell and Douglas Hartmann, "Diversity in Everyday Discourse: The Cultural Ambiguities and Consequences of 'Happy Talk,'" *American Sociological Review* 72, no. 6 (2007): 895.

33. Field note entry, Toward Fair Cures conference, Oakland, California, October 14, 2006.

34. Ibid.

35. Ibid.

36. Ibid.

37. "Induced pluripotent stem cells" (abbreviated as iPS cells) offer the same potential for tissue regeneration that embryonic stem cells do but without the need for embryos. By forcing the expression of particular genes, they can be coaxed in to differentiating.

38. Faden et al., "Public Stem Cell Banks."

39. Ibid.

40. Field note entry, CIRM Diversity Workshop, Charles Drew University of Medicine and Science, Los Angeles, California, February 26, 2010.

41. Durant et al., "Different Types of Distrust."

42. Epstein, "Rise of 'Recruitmentology,'" 816.

43. Hughey, *White Bound*, p. 13.

44. Field note entry, February 10, 2010. This is an excerpt from a behavior contract used at another regional teaching hospital. The nurse who supplied it said that, in her observations, it was "selectively applied" to the predominantly black sickle cell patient population.

45. Field note entry, October 31, 2005, Garvey Research Complex sickle cell clinic.

46. Ibid.

47. Keith Wailoo and Stephen Pemberton, *The Troubled Dream of Genetic Medicine: Ethnicity and Innovation in Tay-Sachs, Cystic Fibrosis, and Sickle Cell Disease* (Baltimore, Md.: Johns Hopkins University Press, 2008).

48. Ibid., 117. This is even more problematic given that such innovations emerge in a broader context of health care deprivation that disproportionately affects African Americans: "Indeed, by the 1990s innovation in sickle cell disease care had come to be seen as a dangerous game—a tricky act of balancing promises of dramatic advances and the perils posted by extraordinary medical experiments against the difficulties of assessing standard medical care" (119).

49. Rayna Rapp, *Testing Women, Testing the Fetus: The Social Impact of Amniocentesis in America* (New York: Routledge, 1999).

50. In many ways, Gaskins exemplifies what Nelson in *Body and Soul* describes as biocultural brokers: individuals or groups who serve as a mediator between Black communities and mainstream medicine.

51. Douglas Lathrop, "The Education of Professir X," *New Mobility,* February 2010, archived at https://web.archive.org/web/20120118232631/http://www.newmobility.com/articleView.cfm?id=11582.

52. Ibid.

53. Gaskin and Young traveled to China to see up close some of Young's clinical trials that use umbilical stem cells and lithium. In Young's words: "This [is] unacceptable. How far have we declined in this country that we have to send people to China to participate in clinical trials of therapies developed in the U.S.? It isn't that umbilical cord blood cells and lithium are at all controversial. The only obstacle is money [to run the trials]." The reality that Americans must engage in medical tourism rather than have access to cutting-edge therapies at home motivates both Young and Gaskin's advocacy and fund-raising.

54. Douglas Lathrop, "Education of Professir X."

55. Michel Callon, "Some Elements of a Sociology of Translation: Domestication of the Scallops and the Fishermen of St. Brieuc Bay," in *Knowledge: Critical Concepts,* ed. Nico Stehr and Reiner Grundmann (New York: Routledge, 2005), 220.

56. Epstein, "Rise of 'Recruitmentology,'" 816.

57. Yancey, Ortega, and Kumanyika, "Effective Recruitment."

58. Epstein, "Rise of 'Recruitmentology,'" 817.

59. Cori Hayden, *When Nature Goes Public: The Making and Unmaking of Bioprospecting in Mexico* (Princeton, N.J.: Princeton University Press, 2003), 21.

60. Eric Lott, *Love and Theft: Blackface Minstrelsy and the American Working Class* (Oxford: Oxford University Press, 1993).

61. "Blackface minstrelsy was an established nineteenth-century theatrical practice, principally of the urban North, in which white men caricatured blacks for sport and profit. It has therefore been summed up by one observer as 'half a century of inurement to the uses of white supremacy.'" Lott, *Love and Theft,* 3.

62. Cheryl I. Harris, "Whiteness as Property," *Harvard Law Review* (1993): 1707–91; Jenny Reardon and Kim TallBear, "Your DNA Is Our History," *Current Anthropology* 53, no. S5 (2012): S235.

63. Ibid., S234.

64. Mary-Jo DelVecchio Good, "The Biotechnical Embrace," *Culture, Medicine, and Psychiatry* 25, no. 4 (2001): 407.

65. Pierre Bourdieu, *The Social Structures of the Economy,* trans. Chris Turner (Cambridge: Polity Press, 2005), 209.

7

Lessons from Racial Medicine
The Group, the Individual, and the Equal Protection Clause

KHIARA M. BRIDGES

In *Adarand Constructors, Inc. v. Peña,* the Supreme Court announced that courts should use strict scrutiny when reviewing laws that contain racial classifications—even those laws that are designed to bring marginalized racial groups into institutions from which they have been historically excluded. Thus, said the Court, "benign" uses of race, like affirmative action programs, would be reviewed with the same skepticism about their constitutionality as "invidious" uses of race.[1] This holding inaugurated the current era of color-blindness in equal protection jurisprudence, wherein the Court treats laws that burden people who historically have enjoyed racial privilege as constitutionally indistinguishable from laws that burden people who historically have not enjoyed racial privilege.[2] The result is that the Court has struck down many laws, including those implementing affirmative action programs, which are designed to benefit racial minorities.

Many color-blind constitutionalists base their opposition to affirmative action on the claim that affirmative action programs are premised on the idea that something is owed to historically subordinated racial groups and that historically privileged racial groups, namely White people, are indebted to people of color. Justice Antonin Scalia, a vocal champion of color-blind constitutionalism, directly disputed this idea of racial indebtedness, writing, "I owe no man anything, nor he me, because of the blood that flows in our veins."[3] Moreover, in his concurrence in *Adarand,* in which the Court struck down a federal affirmative action program in hiring, he wrote:

> In my view, government can never have a "compelling interest" in discriminating on the basis of race in order to "make-up" for past racial

discrimination in the opposite direction. . . . Under our Constitution there can be no such thing as a creditor or debtor race. That concept is alien to the Constitution's focus upon the individual.[4]

Now, it is possible to conceptualize this country's history of racial discrimination as accruing a debt to those racial groups whose contributions to the country—economic, political, cultural, discursive—have been devalued, have gone unrecognized, or have simply been denied. Indeed, it is possible to conceptualize this country's history of racism as compelling state actors to acknowledge that the current subordinate status of racial minorities is a direct result of the debt that is owed to them. In fact, this is how Dr. Martin Luther King Jr. conceptualized the struggle for racial justice. In his 1963 "I Have a Dream" speech, he said:

> In a sense we have come to our nation's capital to cash a check. When the architects of our republic wrote the magnificent words of the Constitution and the Declaration of Independence, they were signing a promissory note to which every American was to fall heir. This note was a promise that all men, yes, black men as well as white men, would be guaranteed the unalienable rights of life, liberty, and the pursuit of happiness. It is obvious today that America has defaulted on this promissory note insofar as her citizens of color are concerned. Instead of honoring this sacred obligation, America has given the Negro people a bad check, a check that has come back marked "insufficient funds." But we refuse to believe that the bank of justice is bankrupt. We refuse to believe that there are insufficient funds in the great vaults of opportunity of this nation. So we have come to cash this check—a check that will give us upon demand the riches of freedom and the security of justice.[5]

If this country's history of racism has created a debt to racial minorities, then affirmative action programs, as a form of reparative or corrective justice, would begin to repay this debt.[6] We would begin to pay off this debt by allowing racial minorities to gain admission to institutions from which they have been excluded historically—acknowledging, albeit belatedly, the contributions that racial minorities have made to this country and putting them in the position where they would have been had the debt never been accrued or had been repaid earlier.

Color-blind constitutionalism denies the debt and thus denies constructing affirmative action programs as a vehicle for repaying it. In denying the debt, color-blind constitutionalists interpret affirmative action programs as grossly illegitimate. Writes Scalia, "The affirmative action system now in place . . . is based upon concepts of racial indebtedness and racial entitlement rather than individual worth and individual need; that is to say, . . . it is racist."[7]

Interestingly, while the Court is increasingly color-blind, biomedical researchers and pharmaceutical companies are seeing color in vivid, and deeply disturbing, ways.[8] These actors are researching, developing, and marketing therapies that are designed to act on the purportedly unique genetic code possessed by distinct racial groups. Here I engage with this species of race-based medicine, which the introduction to this volume describes as "race-targeted pharmaceutical interventions for specific diseases," or ethnopharmacogenomics.

As the introduction explains, ethnopharmacogenomics "considers race and ethnicity to discover if specific genotypes or phenotypes are associated with disease risk and drug response." This form of race-based medicine is one of the most visible hallmarks of the recent reinvigoration of biological race, an idea of race wherein racial groups are imagined to be distinct, genetically homogenous units. The reinvigoration of biological race comes on the heels of more than half century of thought in which it was widely accepted that race is a social construction—a competing idea of race within which racial groups are not products of biological or genetic differences in the human population but rather are biologically arbitrary groupings of humans that are formed as a consequence of political, social, and/or economic forces.[9]

Although ethnopharmacogenomics is based on the false premise that biological race is real—and although engagement with the field might be rejected on that basis alone—the field deserves attention inasmuch as it is a contemporary context in which actors conceive of race as something critical to understanding the individual. Moreover, the field of ethnopharmacogenomics is right in that respect: race *is* critical to understanding the individual, although not for the reasons that ethnopharmacogenomics asserts. Ethnopharmacogenomics claims that race is an important entity that suggests who the individual is in some fundamental, essentialist way, revealing the composition of genes, cells, tissues, enzymes, and so on. In truth, race *is* an important entity that suggests who the individual is in some fundamental way—but not because it exists on the level of an individual's genetic code. It is not *biological* race that suggests who a person is in some fundamental way. Rather, in our racially stratified society, where one's ascribed race predicts and dictates so many aspects of our lives—like where one will live,[10] who one will marry,[11] whether one will marry,[12] whether one will live in poverty,[13] whether one will die while giving birth,[14] whether one's infant will die during birth or shortly thereafter,[15] whether one will be incarcerated,[16] whether one will be sick,[17] and whether one will die earlier than others[18]—it is *socially constructed* race that suggests who a person is in some fundamental way.

Here I engage with ethnopharmacogenomics because the field rightly understands that race is important to understanding the individual, although it misconceives precisely what about race makes it important to understanding the individual. This appreciation of the importance of race to the individual leads the field to deploy the concept in a way that is quite different from the way that race is deployed in modern color-blind equal protection jurisprudence. In so doing, it reveals different possibilities for how race might be deployed in the latter context.

Thus, I analyze and compare how race is used in ethnopharmacogenomics and in equal protection jurisprudence in order to reveal how race is differently conceptualized in these two contexts. Accordingly, I ask: What do ethnopharmacogenomics researchers and pharmaceutical companies believe the nature of race to be? What does race do? What can it reveal? How does it, a group-based characteristic, relate to the individual? The ultimate objective of assessing the use of race in the biomedical context is to ask: What can we learn about how race is implemented within this paradigm? How does it provide a lens through which we can see new things about how race is, and can be, implemented within the equal protection context? Further, what might enthnopharmacogenomics learn from equal protection jurisprudence?

Here I develop two primary insights. First, within the field of ethnopharmacogenomics, race is understood to be a mechanism for accessing the individual in all of her unique particularity. Race is imagined to allow the geneticist, the pharmacogenomics researcher, and the pharmaceutical company to know the individual at her most individual level—at the level of her genotype. Race within this paradigm, then, is thought to be intensely individuating; that is, it is thought to help distinguish an individual from others.[19] However, the geneticist, the pharmacogenomics researcher, and the pharmaceutical company recognize that they can only access an individual's individuality—her genotype—by taking into account her race, a group-based characteristic. Therefore, in the biomedical context, there is no inherent paradox in acknowledging both the individual and the group to which she belongs. Indeed, in this context, in order to treat an individual as an individual, one *must* consider the group to which she belongs—that is, her race. In marked contrast, equal protection jurisprudence regarding affirmative action in recent years has proceeded from the assumption that acknowledging the individual is mutually exclusive to acknowledging the group to which she belongs. The idea within this jurisprudence is that in order to recognize the individual, one must ignore her group. The logical deduction, then, is that recognizing the group necessarily involves ignoring the individual. This theory of the relationship between the individual and the group has led some jurists to conclude that if the Equal Protection Clause demands that the government treat citizens as individuals, then group affiliation (namely the racial group) must be ignored. Ethnopharmacogenomics instructs us that nothing demands this conclusion. Indeed, it instructs us that it is possible to conceptualize group-based characteristics, like race, as being avenues that one must traverse in order to access the individual in her most individual capacity. In essence, the way that race operates in this race-based medicine context helps us to see a potential operation of race that has gone unnoticed in the equal protection context.

Second, this chapter observes that color-blind constitutionalism would lead to striking down most race-conscious laws under the theory that the Equal Protection Clause requires citizens of all races to be treated equally, and equal treatment can only be achieved when state actors do not consciously consider race. As such, color-blind constitutionalism is hostile to the diversity rationale—which *Grutter v. Bollinger* held was a compelling governmental interest, the narrowly tailored pursuit of which will sustain an academic institution's race-conscious admissions program under strict scrutiny review.[20] (The diversity rationale argues that a student body composed of members of diverse racial groups produces educational benefits that a racially homogenous student body cannot replicate. Accordingly, academic institutions may consider race in admissions in order to admit a racially diverse class of students that will generate these educational benefits.) Here I engage with the color-blindness thread in equal protection jurisprudence in order to ascertain how those who author the thread perceive the nature of race in admissions. A close reading of their opinions reveals that jurists writing in this thread are hostile to the use of race in admissions because they view race as inevitably deindividuating. That is, race denies the individuality of the raced individual seeking admission to an academic institution. Of course, this diametrically opposes how race is conceptualized in the field of ethnopharmacogenomics, where geneticists, pharmacogenomics researchers, and pharmaceutical companies consider race to be a means to accessing that which is most individual about a person: her genotype. This is to say that race within ethnopharmacogenomics is imagined to be inherently individuating.[21]

One might reconcile the seemingly different functions of race occurring in the contexts of ethnopharmacogenomics and the Court's affirmative action jurisprudence by theorizing that race operates on two different kinds of mediums in the two contexts. In ethnopharmacogenomics, the medium on which race is operating—the outer surface of the human body—is conceptualized as opaque. The surface of the human body is thought to be opaque because it hides the individuality of the person, comprised as she is of all of her unique allelic variations and genetic sequences. Race, then, is individuating because it purportedly allows third parties to access the individuality hidden within and underneath the body's surface. On the other hand, in the context of the Court's jurisprudence concerning affirmative action in university admissions, the medium on which race is operating is thought to be transparent—the admissions file, which is imagined as allowing third parties to see perfectly and clearly the individuality of the person that the file references. Race, in this context and through this medium, is perceived as deindividuating because it blinds third parties to the other individuating particularities contained within the file, like languages spoken, places traveled, leadership positions held, disadvantages overcome, and unique academic interests pursued. When race is considered in admissions, the argument goes, applicants become deindividuated candidates who are to be admitted, wait-listed, or rejected outright on the basis of their race. I accept this reconciliation and use it as a heuristic for exploring how and why equal protection jurisprudence misapprehends the nature of race.

The heuristic allows one to see that race is thought to be deindividuating when it operates on a transparent surface. It also allows one to see that those who are wary of race-conscious admissions programs conceptualize the admissions file as sufficiently transparent. Accordingly, they think of race as deindividuating. As such, I make the case for race-conscious admissions programs by disputing the assumption that the admissions file is transparent. Instead, if the admissions file—like the outside surface of the human body—is opaque, then race may be understood as individuating. That is, if the admissions file does not actually reveal the individuality of the applicant, then considering the applicant's race may function to further individuate her. Moreover, if race is an individuating mechanism, then being conscious of race is consistent with the contention in *Miller v. Johnson* that the Equal Protection Clause requires the state to "treat citizens as *individuals*, not as simply components of a racial, religious, sexual or national class."[22] Accordingly, I attempt to perform a sort of intellectual jujitsu[23] insofar as I use the weight of the arguments that some have made to oppose affirmative action against the persons making those arguments, thus reformulating anti–affirmative action arguments into those in favor of affirmative action.

Defining Ethnopharmacogenomics

Pharmacogenomics is a branch of pharmacology that attempts to maximize drug efficacy and minimize adverse drug effects by designing pharmaceuticals for specific genotypes.[24] The field of pharmacogenomics is premised on the fact that genes are responsible for the production of enzymes.[25] If a person has a particular gene, it may mean that she produces a particular enzyme that works to metabolize a drug; conversely, if she does not have the gene, it may mean that she cannot produce the particular enzyme that metabolizes a drug. The drug may be toxic or more effective, depending on the presence or absence of the enzyme or gene.[26] The hope of pharmacogenomics is that physicians will know whether to increase or decrease the dosage of a drug, or decline to prescribe it altogether, by looking to whether a patient possesses a specific gene.[27] Pharmacogenomics researchers imagine a utopian future in which drugs will be designed specifically for individuals on the basis of their genetic makeup.[28]

Rapid and affordable mapping of an individual's genetic code is not yet available.[29] Moreover, researchers have yet to develop a drug that has been proven to be more effective for persons possessing specific genes.[30] Thus, we have not arrived at a fully realized era of pharmacogenomics. In the interim, however, race-based medicine, and ethnopharmacogenomics in particular, is offered as the next best thing.[31] As racially profiling doctor Sally Satel explains:

> Doctors look forward to the day when they can, in good conscience, be colorblind. Researchers predict that it will eventually be common practice for doctors to generate a "genomic profile" of every patient—a precise analysis of a person's genetic makeup—so that decisions about therapies can be based on subtle characteristics of the patient's enzyme and receptor biology. At that point, racial profiling by doctors won't be necessary. Until then, however, group identity at least offers a starting point.[32]

Thus, when races are imagined as discrete groups with relative genetic uniformity, a drug or treatment that is designed for an individual's racial group is also designed for an individual's specific genetic code and biology.

The group, race, is a mechanism for accessing the group member's individuality at its most profound, most visceral level. Within the field of ethnopharmacogenomics, race is thus thought to be the best tool at our disposal for making informed assumptions regarding that which is most individual about an individual: her genotype. Far from being an entity that functions to deny a person's particularity, in this particular biomedical context, race is thought to be an entity that makes transparent—through clues apparent on the opaque surface of the human body—an otherwise invisible and practically inaccessible particularity.

The question then becomes, is the admissions file like the surface of the human body? Is it opaque? Or is it transparent, as color-blind constitutionalists believe? Much hinges on the answer to this question. If it is the former, then race might be individuating and its consideration in admissions may be consistent with the Equal Protection Clause's command that persons be treated as individuals, contrary to the assumption made by many who oppose affirmative action. The following section explores the properties of the admissions file.

The Metaphysics of the Admissions File

In an instructive article, Hossler and Kalsbeek identify several models of admissions that guide colleges and universities in the selection of their future student bodies: eligibility-based models, performance-based models, student capacity models, and student capacity to contribute models.[33] While eligibility-based models understand higher education as an entitlement to all prospective students without regard to their performance in their previous educational institutions, performance-based models differ substantially insofar as they "operate with the assumption that admission to college is based upon a meritocracy and that admission is a reward for high performance as well as upon personal characteristics such as perseverance, serving others, and hard work."[34] Performance-based models differ from student capacity models because whereas the former are backward looking, assessing the applicant on the basis of her past performance, the latter do not reward successes that the applicant has already accumulated, instead attempting to "identify talent and to nurture it."[35] Finally, student capacity to contribute models differs from simpler student capacity models because they specifically seek to identify and nurture talent for the labor market.[36]

Save for eligibility-based models, all of the models of admissions that Hossler and Kalsbeek schematize require admissions offices to attempt to get to know who the applicants are as individuals through their applications. With performance-based models, admissions offices essentially conclude that all that is relevant about applicants are their past accomplishments; accordingly, they attempt to get to know applicants by looking at these past accomplishments. In student capacity models, admissions offices assume that applicants are more than the sum total of the successes that they have had in the past; instead, in attempting to divine who the applicants are as individuals, they look to a broader range of activities and experiences—like experiences with poverty or living overseas—in order to identify talent that cannot be identified by the indicia privileged in performance-based models (i.e., standardized test scores and GPAs). Finally, student capacity to contribute models proceeds from the same assumptions as student capacity models while taking a more pragmatic approach to the purpose behind attempting to know the applicants as individuals: they seek to know which individual applicants will be productive workers in the labor force.

Thus, with the exception of eligibility-based models, which tend to be embraced by community colleges and other noncompetitive postsecondary institutions, admissions offices are attempting to get to know who their applicants are through the admissions processes. Unsurprisingly, it is hard to discover who applicants really are as individuals through a process as removed and potentially impersonal as one that involves paper applications. This would explain why there are frequently so many parts to paper applications, including letters of recommendation, personal statements, diversity statements, other writing samples, transcripts from previous educational institutions attended, and reports of scores received on standardized tests. This would also explain why institutions, when they can, supplement the paper admissions process through in-person and phone interviews. All of these are mechanisms through which institutions attempt to get to know applicants as individuals.

If the application process is an endeavor to know applicants in their individual capacities through a woefully deindividuating medium—one that does not allow third parties to clearly see individuals and their particularities and complexities—it would explain the controversy that has surrounded the use of standardized test scores. Standardized testing is offered as a technique through which admissions offices can know that the applicant will do well academically in the institution. The debate around standardized testing is a product of evidence that purports to demonstrate that the results of such testing are better indicators of an individual's group membership than an individual's likelihood of succeeding or failing academically.[37] Accordingly, the charge is that the use of standardized test scores actually impedes an institution's goal of getting to know applicants as individuals. Rather, such testing only provides institutions knowledge of an applicant's family background characteristics (like socioeconomic status, grandparents' socioeconomic statuses, or level of education that parents attained) or relatively insignificant characteristics of an applicant (like the ability to do well on a standardized test that does not accurately predict future performance).[38]

The contention that admissions offices are endeavoring to get to know applicants as individuals via the application process, and that the application is an extremely difficult mechanism through which to get to know applicants as individuals because, despite all of its components, it does not allow third parties to get a sense of an applicant's complexity, is attested to by examining what colleges and universities actually say when explaining to applicants what they are looking for in applications. Consider the following instructions that various schools give to applicants submitting a personal statement, the part of the application that Carbado and Harris describe as an opportunity for applicants "to quite literally inscribe themselves into" the application[39]:

- The personal statement can be the factor that differentiates you from the other candidates. It gives the admissions committee a chance to get a glimpse of you as a person rather than as a set of numbers.[40]
- Be authentic [because the office] want[s] to hear your voice in your response—the experiences, opinions and values that have shaped you. Feel free to write on something you are passionate about so we can get to know you better.[41]
- Please use this opportunity to supply us with any other information that you believe will help us to know you better. This information may be, but is not limited to, a personal history or statement, an explanation of past academic performance, a creative work, a description of an important event in your life or an essay on why you believe you are suited to [the school's] distinctive academic program.[42]
- Your personal essays are the best way for us to learn about you as an individual and to evaluate your academic performance within an appropriate context.[43]
- Numerically, far too many students look identical. It's the intangible pieces: essay, letters of recommendation, and extracurriculars that set one student apart from another.[44]

That the personal statement is supposedly an opportunity for applicants to allow admissions officers to know them as individuals is not unique to the undergraduate context. It is also true in the context of graduate institutions, including law schools. Consider the advice on writing a personal statement that the Law School Admissions Council (LSAC) gives to persons applying to law school:

- Each candidate to law school has something of interest to present. Maybe you've had some experience, some training, or some dream that sets you apart from others. Law schools want to recruit men and women who are qualified for reasons beyond grades and scores. The essay or personal statement in your application is the place to tell the committee about yourself. . . . You are a storyteller here. *You want a living person—you—to emerge. The statement is your opportunity to become vivid and alive to the reader.* (LSAC 2014).[45]

The other parts of an admissions application, beyond the personal statement, can also be understood as attempts by admissions offices to gather information about applicants that will make them into individuals to third-party readers. Consider the website where law school applicants can download LSAC's universal law school application. The LSAC describes letters of recommendation as opportunities for "professors who have known you well enough to write with candor, detail, and objectivity about your academic and personal achievements and potential."[46] Essentially, letters of recommendation are techniques by which third persons give information about a candidate such that a candidate's individuality emerges. Consider also LSAC's description of the "work experience" section of the application: "Law schools want diverse, interesting classes, representative of a variety of backgrounds. A candidate who applies to law school several years after completing his or her undergraduate education, and who has demonstrated an ability to succeed in a nonacademic environment, is sometimes more motivated than one who continues his or her education without a break."[47] Essentially, applicants' descriptions of their work experience provide an opportunity for applicants to give admissions officers yet another facet of their life experience. It is another opportunity for law schools to ascertain the individuality of the person applying for admission.

In sum, the admissions process, at both the undergraduate and graduate levels, is the vehicle through which academic institutions attempt to get to know prospective students as individuals. The purpose of knowing students in this way is multiple: institutions may want to predict whether a student will do well in the institution, whether she has any character flaws or compromised ethics, whether she will contribute to the learning environment in a positive and interesting way, whether she will be a credit to the institution when she is an alumna, and so on. The various elements of an application—GPA, standardized tests scores, personal statements, letters of recommendation, personal interviews when possible—are designed to introduce admissions officers to the actual, living person who submitted the materials. In short, the admissions process is a pursuit toward accessing applicants' individuality.

But there is an important caveat: rankings systems have perverted the admissions process as an endeavor to ascertain the individuality of applicants. For example, the *U.S. News & World Report* rankings of law schools are quite influential, and as a result, they are closely watched by law schools, many of which are well aware that their position in the rankings determines just how coveted seats in the incoming class are—and, ultimately, degrees from the institution.[48] When ranking law schools, *U.S. News & World Report* considers various characteristics, the most important of which is the incoming class's median score on the standardized test all law school applicants take, the Law School Admission Test (LSAT).[49] Accordingly, law schools that are sensitive to the rankings try hard to admit a class whose median is such that the school rises, or at least does not fall, in the rankings. This means that when trying to hit their numbers, schools are most interested in an applicant as an embodiment of an LSAT score. They are less interested in that same applicant as an embodied individual.[50] It is thus entirely accurate to say that the admissions process becomes the opposite of an endeavor to know an applicant as an individual. Instead, it becomes an endeavor to admit standardized test scores that will protect the school's status in the rankings.

There are two important glosses that should be added, however. First, ranking systems pervert the application process as an endeavor to know applicants as individuals only for those institutions for which rankings are significant and that consequently decide to be responsive to them. Second, schools' sensitivity to their incoming classes' median LSAT score does not mean that these are the predominant characteristics that schools consider for all applicants. On the contrary, because the emphasis is on the median (as opposed to the mean), schools are able to admit a significant number of students who have LSAT scores that are lower than the targeted median for the incoming class. As Espeland and Sauder explain:

[U.S. News & World Report] uses the median, the number that cuts the distribution of the LSAT scores and grades in half, rather than the mean in its admissions statistics. The median is more forgiving of outliers in a distribution than the mean. . . . More importantly, the median permits much more latitude since schools can admit students below the median without changing the number too much. Just how many students can be admitted below the median without causing the number to drop depends on the distribution of test scores. In a bell-shaped distribution, more students with lower test scores can be admitted below the median without moving the number much. Some schools take advantage of this statistical bias to admit "whomever we want" below the median.[51]

Thus, the 50th percentile matters—a lot. However, the 1st through 49th percentiles do not matter nearly as much. Accordingly, it is the latter group of applicants, whose numbers are below the score that the institution has targeted for its median, for whom it is most certainly accurate to describe the application process as an endeavor to know the applicant as an individual.

Now, in the past, *U.S. News & World Report* has calculated the median by averaging the scores of the 75th and 25th percentiles of an incoming class.[52] When *U.S. News & World Report* calculates the median in this way, schools care a lot about the scores of their 75th and 25th percentiles. However, scores of the 1st through 25th percentiles do not matter nearly as much. It is this smaller group of applicants, whose numbers are below the score that the institution has targeted for its 25th percentile, for which it is accurate to describe the application process as an endeavor to know the applicant as an individual. For this pool, the question is not whether the applicant's scores will protect the school's place in the rankings; they will not. Instead, the question is, because the applicant cannot protect the school's current place in the rankings with her LSAT scores, what else can she contribute to the institution? It is in this context that law school admissions officers look to the application to reveal whether the applicant is an individual who will be a credit to the school.

With this in mind, I now return to the question, does race facilitate or hinder admissions offices' pursuit of applicants' individuality? This is the question around which the polemic about the consideration of race in university admissions frequently swirls; this is the question that racial medicine in the form of ethnopharmacogenomics could help us answer.

Lessons from Racial Medicine
The Injury of Racial Classifications

The Supreme Court has made it clear that the Equal Protection Clause protects individuals, not groups. Perhaps it is because of the interpretation of the Equal Protection Clause as a defender of the individual that justices, when voting to strike down a racial classification or the use of race in a law, always have at least one eye trained on the harm caused to individuals by the use of race in law. The humanization of the plaintiffs is more than a rhetorical parlor trick; it emphasizes that racial classifications have injured real people.

The question becomes, exactly how have they been injured?[53] What is the injury that these racial classifications have inflicted on them? On one level, the injury is quite specific: the denial of admission to a coveted, competitive college, law school, or medical school. However, coursing beneath and uniting the specific injuries is a general injury: the denial of individuality. Those justices who are most hostile to racial classifications worry about the way that race-conscious laws deny the particularities of individuals and essentialize them, reducing them to just one of their multiplicitous facets: their race.

Race: Individuating or Deindividuating?

The frequently polemical debate about the diversity rationale and its sanctioning of the use of race in university admissions can reasonably be traced to a disagreement about the nature of race. Many who support the diversity rationale and the use of race in admissions conceptualize race as an entity that individuates. Race individuates applicants who are, because of the nature of the application process, deindividuated. These proponents argue that when admissions offices are allowed to know and consider the race of persons submitting applications, they have access to an aspect of the applicant that allows the university to better understand the applicant's uniqueness, making her into a fuller person, as opposed to an accumulation of staid numbers and incomplete stories. In effect, the application may provide a wealth of information about the applicant; however, without knowing the race of the applicant, that information is not enough to let admissions officers fully distinguish the applicant, as an individual, from the host of other applicants with similar information. Race, then, is a mechanism by which the other information provided is placed into context. Thus contextualized, admissions officers can better appreciate who the individual is who presents herself on paper.

In contrast, many who oppose the diversity rationale and the use of race in admissions deny that race is an entity that individuates. Rather, they insist that race operates in exactly the opposite fashion: it is an entity that deindividuates—that essentializes. When admissions offices know and consider the race of persons submitting applications, the consideration thereof renders invisible and/or irrelevant all of the other characteristics of the applicant that make her an individual, like the GPA she earned, scores achieved on standardized tests, extracurricular activities in which she was involved, volunteer work that she has done, special talents she has developed, multiple languages that she speaks, and countries in which she has lived. In effect, many opponents of race-conscious admissions programs contend that the application process successfully allows applicants to present themselves as individuals, and it successfully allows readers of the applications to know the applicants as individuals. However, the consideration of race defeats this feat of individuation, making the applicants into deindividuated persons to be admitted, waitlisted, or rejected outright on the basis of one overriding trait: race.

The First Lesson from Racial Medicine: Why Race Individuates

Ethnopharmacogenomics takes race to be a window into individuality—to an individual genome. Within this paradigm of race, the physician or pharmaceutical company ignores the individuality of the patient when he or it refuses to consider the patient's race. Indeed, when race is not acknowledged, the surface of the body is deindividuating—an opaque medium that hides the individuality of the person, composed as he is of all of his unique allelic variations and genetic sequences. When race is acknowledged, on the other hand, ethnopharmacogenomics believes that the physician and the pharmaceutical company can see through the opacity and view particular aspects of the genotype, that which is most individual about a person. Thus, the philosophy of race that ethnopharmacogenomics embraces finds race, in the absence of better information, to be individuating, and extremely so. (It bears repeating that ethnopharmacogenomics holds race to be individuating at least in part because the field assumes the truth of biological race. Because race is a biological fiction, however, race is not individuating in the way that the field supposes. This does not disqualify the argument. If we substitute the premise of the biological reality of race with that of its social reality, its individuating nature still holds. In this case, race is individuating because it is a social truth that materially and profoundly affects individuals' lives, bodies, and health.)

Ethnopharmacogenomics theorizes that race is individuating when operating on an opaque medium. Therefore, race is individuating in racial medicine because the surface of the human body is thought to be opaque. The question for equal protection jurisprudence becomes, is the admissions file similarly opaque, thereby making race individuating, allowing third parties to see all the particularity contained within it, such as languages spoken, places traveled, leadership positions held, disadvantages overcome, and unique academic interests pursued? Or is the admissions file transparent, thereby making race deindividuating because third parties can already see the particularity contained within it and considering race blinds them to that particularity?

The discussion of the metaphysics of the admissions file above should serve to demonstrate that the answer is the former. The paper application is quite removed and woefully unidimensional—that is, opaque. It does not allow third parties to access the uniqueness of the individual who has submitted the application, even when that application comprises many parts. It is opaque even when it is supplemented by phone or in-person interviews. Thus, race is individuating in admissions because, like racial medicine, it is operating on an opaque medium.

Persons who deploy race as a genetically meaningful category in the development of pharmaceuticals assert that race is an aspect of a person that gets at the truth of individuality in that it serves as a meaningful proxy for genetic code—that which is truly individual. However, because race is a biological fiction, ethnopharmacogenomics errs in this regard. But the field is right in its assertion that race is essential to understanding a person's individuality. This is true for reasons that have nothing to do with biology but have everything to do with the fact that it is a powerful socially constructed marker of access—or lack thereof—to status, resources, safety, and privilege. Race is formative of a person's individuality because in our profoundly racially stratified society, race is a much better predictor of access than it is of one's genetic makeup.

This is absolutely true for those who do not enjoy racial privilege, who tend to be more aware than those with racial privilege about how their racial ascription and identification have shaped the contours of their lives—indeed, about how their race is something that has constituted them as the individuals that they are.[54] But race has also shaped the contours of the lives of those with racial privilege.[55] The difference between those with and without racial privilege may simply be an awareness of the role of race in constituting them in their individualities.

Race is thus an individuating mechanism insofar as it often plays an extensive role in making persons into the individuals they are. It may be that a person's Blackness and the lack of racial privilege that is concomitant with it has made her want to be successful in spite of the odds; as a result, she has become the sum of all of the information that is contained in her application for admission—a speaker of three languages, a classically trained dancer, the valedictorian of her high school, and a writer of spoken-word poetry. It may be that a person's Whiteness and the racial privilege that is concomitant with it has made him aware of the injustice of a country highly stratified by race; as a result, he has become the sum of all of the information that is contained in his application for admission—a speaker of four languages, a community organizer, a political activist, and the valedictorian of his high school.

Many other variations and possibilities exist. It may be that a Black person's class privilege has reduced substantially the effect that her lack of racial privilege would otherwise have had; as a result, she has become the sum of all the information that is contained in her application for admission. It may be that a White person's lack of class privilege has reduced substantially the effect that his racial privilege would otherwise have had; as a result, he has become the sum of all of the information that is contained in his application for admission—a success story despite having attended an underfunded public school, having lived in a neighborhood afflicted with all the problems that afflicts poor neighborhoods, and not having had exposure to the opportunities that those with class privilege have as a matter of course. It may be that a Japanese person's lack of citizenship privilege has substantially reduced the effect that his racial privilege, in some respects, and lack of racial privilege, in other respects, would otherwise have had. It may that a Dominican person's identification as a sexual minority has placed an additional layer of disadvantage on top of her lack of racial privilege. The permutations are endless. Yet the constant in all of the permutations is that race inevitably informs whatever the result is—whatever comprises the compilation of facts, stories, data points, and observations contained in the application for admission.

Thus, race is individuating in the college admissions process. It is individuating not only because it is operating on the opaque medium of the admissions file, but also because it provides context for everything contained in an application for admission. That is, inasmuch as race further illuminates the characteristics that opponents of affirmative action comprehend as individuating, race further individuates individuating characteristics. As a result, race ought to be understood as profoundly individuating. Moreover, if this is what race is, and if admissions offices are engaged in a pursuit to know candidates as individuals, then admissions offices miss a foundational element of every candidate when they fail to consider race. To refuse to see race is to allow every candidate to remain fundamentally unknown.

This argument, of course, depends on the notion that race matters in our society. In order for race to inform the compilation of information contained in every application for admission, race has to matter—and it has to matter for everyone. It is imperative to note that this position does not depend on the assertion that race matters for everyone equally. That is, race does not affect all similarly raced people in the same way. Race does not disadvantage all Black people equally, just as it does not advantage all White people equally. Neither does it ambivalently advantage and disadvantage all non-Black, non-White people equally. An argument that race affects all similarly raced people equally ought to be accused of making problematic—indeed, unconstitutional—generalizations about individuals. Such an argument, when put in practice in an institution's admissions program, certainly deindividuates applicants inasmuch as it assumes a commonality of experience because of a group-based characteristic.

The more nuanced argument here is that race matters in the contemporary United States. Yet the extent to which it has mattered for an individual (how much, in what ways, positively or negatively, and so on) will vary depending on the other characteristics that the individual possesses, such as socioeconomic status, immigration status, citizenship status, sexual orientation, age, gender, and the region of country in which the individual resides. If admissions officers are engaged in an endeavor to know applicants as individuals, then they must consider the nuanced ways that race has intersected with the totality of an individuals' characteristics to produce her as the individual that she is.

The Second Lesson from Racial Medicine: Committing to the Individual While Recognizing the Significance of the Group

Equal protection jurisprudence currently conceptualizes race, a group-based characteristic, as existing in a binary relationship with individuals. Essentially, consideration of the group is mutually exclusive to the consideration of the individual who belongs to the group. Accordingly, to the extent that the group is considered, the individual necessarily goes unconsidered. The corollary to the proposition is that to the extent that the individual is considered, the group must go unconsidered. Because jurists interpret the Equal Protection Clause as demanding that governments treat individuals as individuals, some jurists interpret the clause as prohibiting governmental consideration of the group—that is, of race.

Ethnopharmacogenomics teaches that this philosophy about the nature of the relationship between the group and the individual is deeply flawed. Indeed, the field challenges the supposition that the recognition of the group and recognition of the individual are mutually exclusive, an ontology of race that affirmative action opponents embrace. That is, ethnopharmacogenomics asserts that the group does not necessarily and inevitably exist in a binary relationship to the individual. Persons operating in this field approach individuals' individuality (that is, their individual genome) through acknowledging their group-based characteristic (that is, their race). They claim that recognizing the (racial) group to which an individual belongs is, in the absence of better information, the means to recognizing the individual in his or her most individuated capacity—at the level of the genotype. Accordingly, this species of race-based medicine teaches that we can have a commitment to the individual without rejecting the significance of the group. Indeed, while our ultimate commitment may be to the individual—her need for therapies that work with and respond to her individual genotype—we must simultaneously remain conscious of the group to which she belongs in order to do so. The lesson is that a commitment to the significance of the group and a commitment to the significance of the individual need not be mutually exclusive. Moreover, individuals, the consumers of racial medicine, are told that their group-based characteristics go to the heart of their individuality: when they enter the marketplace of possible therapies for whatever ails them, they must be conscious of their group affiliation if they hope to be treated as individuals.

This is an insight that could have powerful repercussions if recognized in and applied to the context of equal protection. We would first correct ethnopharmacogenomics' misapprehension of race: we would assert that it is not biological race that is formative of persons' individuality, but rather socially constructed race (and its biological repercussions). We would then assert that having a commitment to treating individuals as individuals—a commitment that the Equal Protection Clause might command—does not require that the group (race) lose its significance. As such, the Equal Protection Clause does not demand that race be ignored. On the contrary, governmental actors can be conscious of race while retaining their ultimate commitment to the individual.

But the argument in which racial medicine instructs us—that the Equal Protection Clause *permits* governmental actors to consider race—may not be the strongest argument to which the use of race in ethnopharmacogenomics leads us. Indeed, the use of race in this field may lead us to the conclusion that the Equal Protection Clause *requires* governmental actors to consider race.

Ethnopharmacogenomics teaches us that paying close attention to race can be individuating. The field provides an example of a paradigm within which the only way to treat people as individuals is to take their race into account. What if equal protection jurisprudence operated within the same paradigm? What if the only way to treat people as individuals in admissions was to take their race into account? If the Equal Protection Clause demands that citizens be treated as individuals, and if the only way to treat people as individuals is to take their race into account, then we would arrive at the conclusion that the Equal Protection Clause *obliges* governmental actors to consider race. In this way, ethnopharmacogenomics could turn equal protection jurisprudence on its head—a topsy-turvydom that may be much welcomed by many of those interested in racial justice.

Further, ethnopharmacogenomics argues that individuals, the consumers of medicine, must be conscious of their race because it comprises the heart of their individuality. If an individual hopes to take the anticoagulant that works best for her individual genotype, or to use the therapy for her congestive heart failure that will be most efficacious considering the genes that she possesses, then she must be conscious of her race. Further, she must divulge her race to her health care provider, the person who ultimately facilitates her access to medicine. What if university admissions operated within the same paradigm? If the objective of the admissions process for applicants is to let admissions officers get to know them as individuals, and if an individual's race comprises the heart of their individuality, then individuals applying for admission to institutions would have to be conscious of their race if they hoped to allow admissions officers to get to know them fully as individuals. Additionally, they would have to divulge their races to admissions officers, the persons who ultimately facilitate their access to institutions (by accepting the applicant). The significance of this is that ethnopharmacogenomics suggests that the personal statement would not be a tool that racial minorities use to tell stories about how their racial identification or ascription has affected their lives. Instead, it would be a tool that all persons would use to tell stories about how their race has worked to produce them as the individuals that they are. It would compel White people—who frequently are unaware of the benefits that their racial ascription brings—to contemplate how their race has advantaged them in innumerable ways. If the racial privilege that White people experience is owed in part to the invisibility of Whiteness, then compelling White persons to be conscious of their race is a much-needed first step in the dismantling of this privilege.

Conclusion
Lessons from Equal Protection Jurisprudence

I have argued that equal protection jurisprudence can learn a few things from race-based medicine, specifically ethnopharmacogenomics. The question then becomes, can race-based medicine learn anything from equal protection jurisprudence? The answer is yes.

At the time of this writing, affirmative action programs are consistent with the mandates of the Equal Protection Clause. In *Grutter v. Bollinger*, a majority of the Supreme Court held that although affirmative action programs are constitutionally suspect and must be subjected to the most vigorous judicial scrutiny, courts should uphold them if such programs are a pursuit of the educational benefits that a "diverse" student body purportedly produces. (The Court affirmed the legitimacy of the diversity rationale when it reviewed the Fifth Circuit's approval of race consciousness in undergraduate admissions at the University of Texas in *Fisher v. Texas II*.[56]) However, the diversity rationale might be the most disturbing part of *Grutter*. The reign of the diversity rationale came on the heels of the death of the "remedying past societal discrimination" rationale. That is, while the pursuit of a diverse student body could save an affirmative action program from unconstitutionality after *Grutter*, the earlier jurisprudence had established that the attempt to remedy past societal discrimination could not save such a program. While the end is the same (more racial minorities gain access to schools that otherwise would be inaccessible), the means to the end are troubling. Why is "diversity" more constitutionally attractive than "remedying past societal discrimination"? The answer may be that those who are imagined to benefit from programs designed to remedy past societal discrimination are only the minority groups that were victims of discrimination; however, those who are imagined to benefit from programs designed to increase diversity include nonminorities. To be clear, the programs are the same. But when "diversity" is the justification for the program, it allows us to imagine that even White people benefit. Both non-White people and White people acquire cross-racial understanding. Both non-White people and White people are disabused of racial stereotypes. Both non-White people and White people are prepared to enter a multicultural workforce. There may be some losers with diversity, namely White (and Asian) applicants who are denied admission under a race-conscious admissions program and who may have been admitted if the university had a race-blind program. However, most importantly, White people—specifically those White people who are present in the classroom with racial minorities—are winners too.

While it is likely true that individuals of all racial ascriptions and identifications benefit from racially diverse environments, it is concerning that when the interest was framed in terms that focused only on the benefit that minorities would receive from affirmative action—when it was articulated in the language of "remedying past societal discrimination"—a majority of the Supreme Court refused to find that this interest was compelling. That is, a majority of the Court refused to recognize how compelling it was for the state to rectify the enduring effects of the mistreatment, disenfranchisement, and denial of citizenship experienced by racial minorities in the United States. A majority of the Court refused to recognize that that this country owes a debt to historically marginalized racial groups—groups whose marginalization has provided unquantifiable (and uncompensated) benefits to racial groups with privilege. The Court denied this country's indebtedness. It denied conceptualizing affirmative action as a form of reparative justice (i.e., repaying what is owed to the creditor). This denial impoverishes the discourse around affirmative action as well as the programs themselves. It allows us to pretend, quite dangerously, that our history does not affect our present. Race-based medicine might learn from this. It might learn that it risks impoverishment when it denies that present health states and health disparities are informed by this country's past.

It is worth asking what race-based medicine would look like if it truly were a form of reparative justice. What shape would it take if it was pursued from a position that recognized that our history impacts our present? What if it was interested in addressing that lamentable history such that the injustices that were made in the past would not have continuing effects in the present? While there may be several directions in which race-based medicine could go if it were a project of reparative justice, it most certainly would not go in the direction of ethnopharmacogenomics.

Ethnopharmacogenomics repairs nothing. It locates the causes of racial disparities in health in the genes, as opposed to the social structures within which individuals exist—the structures that actually influence whether or not someone will have hypertension, asthma, diabetes, or certain types of cancer. It denies that our history of racial disenfranchisement has effects on individuals' present health states. Indeed, ethnopharmacogenomics rejects claims of past wrongs, but then it attempts to remedy the effects of those wrongs by pointing to individual "genetic" deficits. In actuality, if race-based medicine were pursued as a form of reparative justice, it would hold within its field of vision housing, the social safety net, voting, mass incarceration, immigration policy, the criminalization of property crimes, and a wealth of other areas that affect whether people are sick or healthy, whether they live or die.

Nevertheless, many see race-based medicine, as presently constituted, as a way of repaying America's debt to racial minorities by attempting to undo some of the lasting physical toll this debt has taken on their bodies. They see ethnopharmacogenomics as the most promising and effective avenue for reducing racial health disparities. However, if race is a social construct that produces poorer health outcomes and risk profiles for some groups, as opposed to a collection of genes that can be "corrected for" and thereby produce better health outcomes, then this line of repayment amounts to "a check that has come back marked 'insufficient funds.'"

Notes

1. *Adarand Constructors Inc. v. Peña*, 515 U.S. 200, 227 (1995).
2. Some Supreme Court justices deny that we have entered an era of colorblindness in equal protection jurisprudence. For example, in *Parents Involved in Community Schools v. Seattle School District No. 1*, Justice Breyer said in dissent, "I can find no case in which this Court has followed Justice Thomas' 'color-blind' approach." 557 U.S. 701, 832–33 (2007). Moreover, a majority of the justices currently sitting on the Supreme Court have not affirmed the contention that the Equal Protection Clause requires color-blindness. This is evidenced by Justice Kennedy's opinion in the same case noting that Justice Harlan's assertion in his *Plessy* dissent that the Constitution is color-blind must "as an aspiration, . . . command our assent . . . [yet,] in the real world, it is regrettable to say, it cannot be a universal constitutional principle" (788).
3. Antonin Scalia, "The Disease as Cure: 'In Order to Get Beyond Racism, We Must First Take Account of Race,'" *Washington University Law Review* 1979 (1979): 153.

4. *Adarand Constructors Inc. v. Peña*, 515 U.S. 200 (1995), 239.
5. Martin Luther King Jr., "I Have a Dream," https://www.archives.gov/files/press/exhibits/dream-speech.pdf.
6. Kimberlé Crenshaw, "The Court's Denial of Racial Societal Debt," *Human Rights* 40 (2013): 12–14, 16.
7. Scalia, "Disease as Cure," 154.
8. On its face, it is somewhat ironic that the Court is embracing color-blindness within constitutional law while biomedicine is embracing color-consciousness within pharmaceutical research. However, Dorothy Roberts has argued that it is actually consistent that the Court has refused to see race while biomedicine has insisted on seeing it. Roberts, "Legal Constraints on the Use of Race in Biomedical Research: Toward a Social Justice Framework," *Journal of Law, Medicine, and Ethics* 34 (2006): 526–34. She observes that advocates of color-blindness in constitutional law frequently assert that the problem of racism is over and that we now exist in a postracial era. However, it is undeniable that this purported postracial era is rife with stratification along racial lines. She contends that racial difference at the biological level helpfully explains continued social inequalities between racial groups. "Biological distinctions, seemingly validated by genomic science and technology, appear to explain why stark racial disparities persist despite the abolition of official discrimination on the basis of race and despite [some] Americans' belief that racism has ceased to exist." Roberts, *Fatal Invention: How Science, Politics, and Big Business Re-create Race in the Twenty-first Century* (New York: New Press, 2011), 297. As such, Roberts views color-blindness within constitutional law and color-consciousness within biomedicine as consistent because if racism is over (as many advocates of constitutional color-blindness contend), then the fact that, for example, maternal mortality rates for Black mothers are almost four times those of White mothers, and racial minorities, specifically Black people, die younger than White people in the United States, must be explained in terms of genetic differences between races and not in terms of structural racism. T. J. Matthews and Marian F. MacDorman, "Infant Mortality Statistics from the 2008 Period Linked Birth/Infant Death Data Set," *National Vital Statistics Report* 60, no. 5 (2010): 1–27.
9. Kamala Visweswaran, "Race and the Culture of Anthropology," *American Anthropologist* 100, no. 1 (1998): 70–83.
10. Lincoln Quillian, "Segregation and Poverty Concentration: The Role of Three Segregations," *American Sociology Review* 77 (2012): 354–79.
11. Wendy Wang, "The Rise of Intermarriage: Rates, Characteristics Vary by Race and Gender," *Pew Research Center, Social and Demographic Trends*, February 16, 2012, http://www.pewsocialtrends.org/files/2012/02/SDT-Intermarriage-II.pdf.
12. Richard R. Banks, *Is Marriage for White People? How the African American Marriage Decline Effects Everyone* (New York: Penguin, 2011).

13. "Poverty in the United States: Frequently Asked Questions," *National Poverty Center*, http://www.npc.umich.edu/.

14. "Births, Deaths, Marriages, and Divorces," in "Statistical Abstract of the United States," U.S. *Bureau of the Census*, August 2011, http://www.census.gov/prod/2011pubs/12statab/vitstat.pdf.

15. Cheryl Lipscomb and Marci Lobel, "Explaining Disproportionately High Rates of Adverse Birth Outcomes among African Americans: The Impact of Stress, Racism, and Related Factors in Pregnancy," *Psychology Bulletin* 131 (2005): 662.

16. Marc Mauer, "Addressing Racial Disparities in Incarceration," *Prison Journal* 91 (2011): 88S.

17. Margaret T. Hicken, "A Novel Look at Racial Health Disparities: The Interaction between Social Disadvantage and Environmental Health," *American Journal of Public Health* 102 (2012): 2344–51.

18. Patrick M. Krueger, Jarron M. Saint Onge, and Virginia W. Chang, "Race/Ethnic Differences in Adult Mortality: The Role of Perceived Stress and Health Behaviors," *Social Science and Medicine* 73 (2012): 1313.

19. To be more precise, race within biomedicine aspires to be individuating to the point where race no longer matters—that is, we have arrived at the era of personalized medicine. But in the meantime, the use of race individuates to the extent that the group membership is seen as predictive of individual outcomes.

20. *Grutter v. Bollinger*, 539 U.S. 306 (2003).

21. Of course, ethnopharmacogenomics makes the argument that race—biological race, to be precise—is individuating. However, because biological race is a myth and race is not biological fact, the assumption that individuals have certain genotypical features by mere dint of their social grouping is in fact deindividuating.

22. *Miller v. Johnson*, 515 U.S. 900, 911 (1995).

23. Thanks to Jonathan Khan for colorfully, and flatteringly, using this phrase to describe this chapter.

24. Osagie K. Obasogie, "The Return of Biological Race? Regulating Innovations in Race and Genetics through Administrative Agency Race Impact Statements," *Southern California Interdisciplinary Law Journal* 22, no. 1 (2012): 1–64.

25. Liam Drew, "Pharmacogenetics: The Right Drug For You," *Nature* 537 (2016): S60–S62.

26. Ibid.

27. Ibid.

28. Roberts, *Fatal Invention*.

29. John Lauerman, "Complete Genomics Drives Down Cost of Genome Sequence to $5,000," *Bloomberg*, February 5, 2009, archived at http://web.archive.org/web/20121023234539/http://www.bloomberg.com/apps/news?pid=newsarchive&sid=aEUlnq6ltPpQ.

30. However, there have been optimistic developments on this front. With respect to leukemia, researchers have been able to identify a gene that correlates with drug toxicity; patients can be tested for the gene, and the results of the test will determine the course of treatment. Erika L. Moen, Lucy A. Godley, Wei Zhang, and M. Eileen Dolan, "Pharmacogenomics of Chemotherapeutic Susceptibility and Toxicity," *Genome Medicine* 4 (2012): 90. Similar advances have been made in breast cancer research. Sarah C. P. Williams, "Genetics to Determine Cancer Treatment," *Los Angeles Times*, September 13, 2012, http://articles.latimes.com/.

31. William E. Evans and Mary Relling, "Pharmacogenetics: Translating Functional Genomics into Rational Therapies," *Science* 286 (1990): 487–91.

32. Sally Satel, "I Am a Racially Profiling Doctor," *New York Times*, May 5, 2002, http://www.nytimes.com/.

33. Don Hossler and David Kalsbeek, "Admissions Testing and Institutional Admissions Processes: The Search for Transparency and Fairness," *College and University*, 84, no. 4 (2009): 4.

34. Ibid.
35. Ibid.
36. Ibid.
37. Ibid.

38. Lani Guinier, "Admissions Rituals as Political Acts: Guardians at the Gates of Our Democratic Ideals," *Harvard Law Review* 117 (2003): 113–224.

39. Devon W. Carbado and Cheryl I. Harris, "The New Racial Preferences," *California Law Review* 96 (2008): 1144.

40. Ibid.
41. Ibid., 1183.

42. Undergraduate Admissions, "Personal Statement/Essay," *Worcester Polytechnic Institute*, archived at https://web.archive.org/web/20131004053321/http://www.wpi.edu/admissions/undergraduate/apply/essay.html.

43. "Personal Essay Questions: Undergraduate Admission Application," *University of Colorado, Boulder*, archived at https://web.archive.org/web/20140612001403/http://www.colorado.edu/sites/default/files/attached-files/Personal_essays.pdf.

44. "Writing a Personal Statement," *Vanderbilt University Undergraduate Admissions*, September 30, 2010, http://admissions.vanderbilt.edu/.

45. One could claim that these descriptions of the personal statement might be driven more by how institutions want to be perceived by outsiders rather than by what institutions believe the goal of personal statements—and admissions generally—to be. However, the reality is that admissions committees and the members that compose them are charged with the duty to admit a class of persons that the institution wants to count as students—and eventually alumni. To this end, admissions officers read the personal statement contained in each application that needs to be reviewed. It is important to note that they are reading personal

statements written by persons who have been told that such statements are opportunities for themselves as "living persons . . . to emerge"—opportunities to make themselves less identical to the hordes of other applicants. It is also important to note that for most institutions, especially the more elite ones, the number of applications that they receive dwarfs the number of seats available for the incoming class. "Applying to Law School: How Law Schools Determine Whom to Admit," *Law School Admissions Counsel,* 2014, http://www.lsac.org/. As such, it is not unreasonable to assume that, even if the above descriptions of the personal statement might be understood cynically as efforts made by institutions to present a certain facade, admissions officers end up knowing a lot about an applicant as an individual after reading the intentionally personal information contained in the submitted statements. Moreover, it is not unreasonable to assume that admissions officers end up sympathizing with, thinking more highly of, and being more inclined to admit applicants who have managed to provide glimpses of themselves as individuals in the personal statement, thus distinguishing themselves from the pool of qualified applicants fighting for seats that are in limited supply. Getting to know the applicant as an individual thus becomes folded within the application process, whether or not the institution intended for that to be a goal.

46. Ibid.
47. Ibid.
48. Michael Sauder and Wendy Espeland, "Fear of Falling: The Effects of *U.S. News & World Report* Rankings on U.S. Law Schools," *LSAC Research Report Series,* October 2007, http://www.lsac.org/docs/default-source/research-%28lsac-resources%29/gr-07-02.pdf.
49. Ibid.
50. One can find numerous examples of how the singular focus on the LSAT has perverted the admissions process. Espeland and Sauder quote an administrator as saying, "The dean will say to the admissions director, 'I want a 160.' And I've had admissions directors tell me that. 'I have been instructed to produce X if at all possible.' Well, that tells you what their admissions process is going to be like." Wendy N. Espeland and Michael Sauder, "Fear of Falling: The Influence of Media Rankings on Legal Education in America," February 2012, http://www.law.berkeley.edu/files/csls/Paper_-_Espeland.doc, 10. They quote another admissions director as saying, "The University of Toledo does a symposium every year where they have deans come in and they give the status of the academy, and I have lots of quotes of people saying that they had to choose between a person with a 160 and a 3.5 and a person with a 170 and a 2.2. Well, the 160 won't help you in the *[U.S. News & World Report]* ranking but the 170 will. But, realistically, you think that the person with the 160 and 3.5 is more likely to succeed, but they are gaming the rankings so the 170 person gets in. It happens all the time" (10).
51. Ibid., 38.

52. Jeffrey E. Stake, "The Interplay between Law School Rankings, Reputations, and Resource Allocation: Ways Rankings Mislead," *Indiana Law Journal* 81 (2008): 229–70.

53. There is a strong argument to be made that White persons who do not gain admission to educational institutions because of affirmative action programs had not been injured at all. This argument contends that individuals are injured by racial classifications only when the racial classification functions to stigmatize them as inferior. Take, for example, Justice Brennan's opinion in *Regents of the University of California v. Bakke,* where he contends that the "cardinal principle" of the Equal Protection Clause is that "racial classifications that stigmatize—because they are drawn on the presumption that one race is inferior to another or because they put the weight of government behind racial hatred and separatism—are invalid without more." 438 U.S. 265 (1978).

54. Darren Lenard Hutchinson, "Progressive Race Blindness? Individual Identity, Group Politics, and Reform," *UCLA Law Review* 49 (2001–2): 1455–80.

55. Jerry V. Diller, *Cultural Diversity: A Primer for the Human Services* (Belmont, Calif.: Brooks/Cole, 2011), 54.

56. Linda Greenhouse, "The Supreme Court's Diversity Dilemma," *New York Times*, December 24, 2015, http://www.nytimes.com/.

CONCLUSION

Freedom from Debt?

LESLIE R. HINKSON AND NADINE EHLERS

Through framing race as biological and as the underlying cause of health disparities, architects of race-based medicine have laid the groundwork for a tripartite system of health care delivery, biomedical practice, and biomedical research that has simultaneously racialized disease and illness and rationed access to and quality of care along racial lines. This system has created a space for health disparities—rooted in slavery, settler colonialism, Jim Crow, and residential segregation—to grow, and for health-related costs and debt to accumulate to its victims. Such debts, as the chapters collected here explore, impose a financial toll in addition to emotional, psychological, and social costs. Several contributions in this volume have illustrated how race-based medicine has created monetary debts for minority subjects through limited access to affordable care and through a history of social and medical abuse and neglect that created health disparities. These disparities are costly to address—in pure monetary terms—and such costs are often squarely placed on the shoulders of racial minorities themselves. Additionally, race-based medicine has, in recent decades, augmented the creation of debt through the formulation of race-targeted treatments that are associated with larger price tags than those used to treat nonminority subjects with similar ailments.

Are the terms of repayment any less onerous when the debt is conceived as a moral as opposed to a monetary one? In other words, does the United States as a whole suffer emotionally, financially, psychologically, and socially as a result of the moral or ethical debt burden associated with its historical role in helping to both create and maintain disparities in the health profiles of racial minorities compared with their White counterparts? The contributions of this volume suggest that it does. As many authors in this volume argue, race-based medicine today is often positioned as an attempt to redeem the nation's less than virtuous past: it is framed as a means through which we might redress past injuries and repay this accumulated debt. However, race-based medicine often fails to address the conditions that created this debt in the first place, and rather than serving to defray that debt and alleviate attendant suffering, it often functions to maintain the status quo and thus entrench past injury.

An enduring question that remains is, what are the problematics of framing race-based medicine as an adequate or even appropriate form of redress? Rather than ensuring that all people have access to affordable, healthy food, for example, we provide them with race-targeted pharmaceutical treatments for hypertension and diabetes. Rather than pouring more resources into studying the social and environmental determinants of breast cancer, we invest more heavily in the search for race-specific genetic factors to explain the increased likelihood of African American women dying from the disease than their White counterparts. Rather than investing in increasing the supply of affordable, quality health care in minority communities, particularly where the inhabitants are lower income, we expand Medicaid coverage. But what use is health insurance if the health providers you are able to access view your coverage as inferior to other forms and so won't accept it? Or, what if those providers don't offer quality care, or are too few in number to serve everyone in the community requiring their services?

Ultimately, such approaches all come with significant monetary costs, and all attempt to address health disparities in some way. Some have even been specifically crafted as a means of social redress for the existence of these disparities. However, none truly focuses on eliminating them. Thus, race-based medicine can be seen as a racial project that, in our contemporary era, is greatly influenced by the tenets of neoliberalism: it extends a meaning of race based in biology—which is used to rationalize the organization and distribution of both medical services and medical knowledge—without disrupting profit margins or shareholder value.[1] Indeed, it yields the future promise of both better health outcomes for those who fall under the racialized biomedical gaze and greater wealth to those invested in its many forms of expansion. To date, however, wealth associated with race-based medicine has only accrued to a select few, and as the cost of health care rises, minorities continue to experience excessive rates of morbidity and mortality. Thus, the specter of guilt recursively haunts the conscience of the nation, and that guilt continues to keep the United States a nation divided.

In examining race-based medicine through the lens of debt, the chapters in this volume return again and again to its main limitation: its rationalization and practice reveal a poor theorization of race. That race should be conceptualized as a biological reality, or even an admittedly crude yet necessary stand-in for genetic variation, reveals an underdeveloped and ahistorical understanding of the concept's past and present as a sociopolitical category. In a form of teleological reasoning, race becomes an explanatory variable—the supposed cause of racial health disparities—without much attention being placed on what race is or the casual mechanisms and pathways through which race operates as a predictor of health profiles. Such reasoning is indicative of a disturbing trend in biomedicine that may well disseminate across the rest of society: the reentrenchment of race as biological "truth" in a field that is esteemed as a hard science, whose assumptions are in many ways seen as inviolable by many other academic disciplines and by the public, may serve to not only provide biological explanations for health and other racial disparities found in our society but to provide justification for them as well.

The reentrenchment of the idea that race is biological makes for poor science. To be clear, it is to be expected that medical practitioners and researchers should focus on the body, on the biological roots of disease, and on the biological responses to external stimuli. The problem with race-based medicine, particularly as it relates to ethnopharmacology, is not that it focuses on the biological but in that it treats race as a possible biological determinant or root cause/trigger of disease as opposed to thinking of race as predicting the amount of exposure to a series of external stimuli that invoke certain biological responses. For example, African Americans are more likely to be diagnosed with nitric oxide deficiency than Whites. This condition can be caused by obesity, stress, diet, and lack of exercise, among other factors. In other words, the primary causes are external to the individual. Yet scores of scientific and medical journals recommend, given the higher probability of nitric oxide deficiency in this population, that beta-blockers are not an effective alternative pharmaceutical option when considering treatment for hypertension or congestive heart failure. If this deficiency is what explains the lack of effectiveness of the drug in individuals, why not simply test all patients with hypertension or congestive heart failure for nitric oxide deficiency in order to determine the best course of treatment? Why simply use race—whether self-identified or assumed by the health care professional—as a proxy for a specific biological process? In focusing on the racial category as opposed to low levels of nitric oxide, the former becomes the focus of treatment, the deficiency to be overcome. Biomedicine, we would suggest, needs to focus more on what is broken in bodies and the pathologies to be found in biological processes, rather than biologizing what is broken and pathological in our society.

A primary purpose of this volume has been to reveal the hidden costs of race-based medicine and the flawed logics that undergird it by showing its association with debt. A second but no less important goal has been to begin articulating alternative ways of approaching health disparities—and wellness more broadly—for minorities in the United States. Such alternative means would necessarily be based in sound science and not stereotypes, and they would recognize (contrary to the belief of many) that the existing U.S. health care system already rations care.[2] This rationing plays a role in the amount of care people have access to and in how medical practitioners and researchers alike conceptualize the qualitative aspects of that care. The overriding question that surely must structure any future direction would be, how do we address racial disparities in health—that is, acknowledging the rationing of care and the rationalization of underserving certain racialized individuals and communities—without running into the danger of reinstantiating notions of race as biological truth or destiny? In response, three major themes on how to begin rethinking and even replacing race-based medicine are repeated across many of the contributions in this volume.

The first theme advanced is that increased attention must be paid—in both biomedical care and research—to the structural and social determinants of health disparities specifically and to wellness more generally. Nadine Ehlers and Shiloh Krupar, for instance, illustrate how medical hot spotting shifts the focus away from the structural determinants of health and onto the behaviors and culture of those whose health has been compromised by larger systems of social inequality. In placing the responsibility of reducing medical costs and health disparities on the shoulders of patients and medical practitioners, we run the risk of both augmenting racial inequality and of further reifying race as a biological fact, re-securing the erroneous message that certain racial groups enjoy poorer health not because of external forces but because of deficits, biological or cultural, seen as inherent to the group itself. Jenna Loyd shows how the framing of the congressional debate over the passage of the Affordable Care Act evaded discussion of race, effectively obscuring the relationship between universal health care and the past and present harms of structural racism such that it is almost entirely erased from public discourse. In ignoring how the sociopolitical origins of racial classification in the

United States and its history of structured inequality come together to create health disparities, we effectively excise the main determinants of health inequality. In papering over discussions of the structural and social determinants of health, particularly as it relates to race, legislators and policy makers can downplay the nation's ethical responsibility to provide health care to all—a policy that would be a good and necessary step toward effectively addressing many of the inequalities embedded within the economy, the political process, and the social fabric at large.

Furthering this theme, Anne Pollock asserts that the focus on BiDil, or any one pill (whether to assess the monetary costs associated with race-based medicine or to try to reduce disparities in the prevalence of congestive heart failure), is a distraction: it blinds us to broader operations of marginalization within the nation's racially fragmented system of health care delivery and medicine. Rather than becoming preoccupied with monetary costs of the physical pill at the pharmacy, we must examine the range of costs associated with obtaining a prescription in the first place. And rather than simply focusing on and investing in treating disease, we should be paying more attention to environmental, political, and social factors that contribute to higher levels of the incidence of congestive heart failure in certain populations—an approach to addressing health disparities that goes well beyond assumed micro-level biological differences. Catherine Bliss cautions against the growing trend in health disparities research that places priority on sociogenomic projects that do little to incorporate the social in their inquiry. This threatens to solidify biological notions of race within the entire scientific community and impedes progress in finding truly effective means of reducing health disparities. Finally, Ruha Benjamin and Leslie Hinkson illustrate how the lack of attention to the history behind why certain groups are less likely to enroll into clinical trials hinders the efforts of researchers to effectively recruit them and leads to the reification of race as a marker of inherent deficits in desired cultural traits. In order to truly achieve the goal of inclusion in clinical trials, recruiters need to place more focus on the past practices of the biomedical establishment that created the lack of trust in the institution in the first place, as well as the current practices that do little to earn trust from prospective minority recruits and their broader communities today.

Viewed through the lens of the five chapters referenced above, paying greater attention to the social and structural determinants of health would not only radically improve the quality of the work being done to reduce health disparities but would also hold more potential for improving the overall health of racial minorities specifically and U.S. national health generally. Increasing the focus in this direction would not preclude investment in research at the genomic level, but it would challenge research that treats race as a marker of biological difference as opposed to a socially constructed marker of differential access to status, power, and a range of resources needed to support favorable health outcomes. How, then, might we ensure that greater attention is given to the social determinants of health in systems of health care delivery, medical care, and biomedical research? First, we suggest that an initial step would be to change the funding priorities of major grant-awarding agencies, including those for research as well as those for health- and medical-related services. Researchers and service organizations craft their projects and programs to meet the priorities set by the funders' requests for proposals. If grantor organizations provided more funding for projects and programs that either focused specifically on the economic, sociological, and political factors that affect health outcomes or that incorporated these factors more effectively in genome-based ones, the way that race is used in research and to design health-related services would begin to follow suit. Second, PhD programs in the various biomedical fields could train future researchers and practitioners in the importance of these structural and social determinants of health as a means of complementing their training on the genetic components of disease and illness. Medical schools and doctor training programs could follow suit, instructing future doctors in the appropriate use of race in the biomedical encounter—not as a data point to dictate specific diagnoses or treatment regimens based primarily on population-level risk profiles, but as a factor to help contextualize individuals and their medical needs when information on things such as family medical history, present living conditions, and individual-level medical information are unavailable.[3]

A second theme presented regarding how race-based medicine might be rethought or replaced is by a radical revision—in both biomedical care and research—of how race itself is conceptualized and understood to operate. Leslie Hinkson notes that race is often used as a shortcut for inferring differences in a drug's effectiveness in patients. Such inferences often lead to treatment decisions that go against established medical guidelines and may be ineffective. Because race in this instance is used as a true marker of biological difference, doctors will potentially withhold treatment regimens that are both the most medically appropriate and perhaps the most cost effective. Catherine Bliss states, "Notions of race and health disparities have been increasingly biologized," and as a result, "redress for social inequality has been reenvisioned in the form of pills and diagnostics." In conceptualizing race and its related forms of inequality as biological in nature, our society risks allowing these inequalities to become exacerbated, both because of the failure to address their real causes and because such a formulation in the hard sciences and biomedicine pose the danger of disseminating into other areas of society. This was seen, for example, a little over twenty years ago, when Herrnstein and Murray's *The Bell Curve* (1994) reignited old debates about the genetic basis of intelligence and of race. The widely circulated text argued that, given both were heritable, the gap in the average IQ scores between Whites and Blacks was clearly genetic in nature.[4] Thus, it was claimed, no amount of spending or attention to curriculum would help to decrease the deficiencies in intelligence found in the latter group. Race-based medicine's formulation of race as biological—or at the very least as a stand-in for legitimate biological processes—opens the door to, and indeed invites a reinvigoration of, arguments like those found in *The Bell Curve* in fields as seemingly disparate as banking (access to capital), criminal justice, education, and employment.

Extending this theme, Ruha Benjamin and Leslie Hinkson's chapter highlights the way that race is often conceptualized as an innate cultural disposition, causing some groups to have more or less trust in medicine, especially when it comes to enrollment into clinical trials. Rather than seeing the level of trust that certain communities hold in the biomedical enterprise as rational responses to historical patterns of harm, it is conceptualized as an intrinsic cultural attribute. Such a reification of race serves to undermine the recruitment of minorities in clinical trials and at times to maintain a culture within biomedicine that continues to hold the threat of future exploitation. Khiara Bridges, in her articulation of the connections between race-based medicine and equal protection jurisprudence, concludes that the former's conceptualization of race as revealing some hidden "truth" about an individual's genetic makeup misapprehends the nature of race itself. In so doing, the practitioners of race-based medicine (in this case, ethnopharmacogenomics) risk moving away from the goal of individualized medicine and toward one in which racial profiles play an outsized role in the research and treatment of members of minority groups.

In the four chapters referenced above, the authors note how problematic conceptualizations of race—whether as genetically based or as evidence of innate cultural dispositions—serve to undermine the stated goals of those who use them to inform their research or their approach to medical treatment. How, then, might a significant paradigmatic shift in how race is used and conceptualized in biomedicine be achieved? In one sense, individuals both within and outside of biomedical fields need to push our colleagues to not just state how they conceptualize race in their research and practice but also to justify that conceptualization in addition to the very use of race itself. There are instances of publications in leading medical and public health journals where individuals and groups of researchers have banded together to question the proper use of race in biomedicine and biomedical research.[5] Such efforts are necessary, but they are also few and far between. Social science scholars must do their part as well. For all of the rhetoric concerning the socially constructed nature of race, too few that focus on race-related research—be it in biomedicine, health, or other fields—take adequate care in conceptualizing race. Merely operationalizing race in terms of standard U.S. categories is not enough. Why is race used in their studies, and how is it used? Even more rare is the social scientist who focuses on directly examining or illustrating the ways racial categories are not tied to meaningful biological differences. Rather than proving to themselves over and over in their own journals that race is a social construction, why not attempt to publish more in biomedical journals and directly dispute racial essentialism or biologization, using the language of the readers of those journals? Dismantling the idea of race as inherent will take collaboration across disciplines and a willingness for each of us to in effect "discipline our disciplines"—to take better care with the use of this highly volatile concept. In another and related sense, more serious research needs to be conducted with race as the primary subject of inquiry, as opposed to a control variable or an explanatory variable that is not sufficiently vetted as a legitimate causal factor. If editorial boards, anonymous reviewers, and funding organizations held researchers to these standards, the entire knowledge production process would begin to shift toward more appropriate definitions and uses of race in publishing, in research, and ultimately in practice and service provision.

A final theme the authors present is how to begin revising past and present incarnations of race-based medicine to extend the goal of inclusion beyond biomedical research—to incorporate broader access to care and the resources to maintain or aspire to wellness. Inclusion could be pursued not simply for the sake of diversity alone nor for the primary benefit of biomedicine, but for the sake of health itself. Anne Pollock notes that many applauded the actions of the U.S. Food and Drug Administration to approve BiDil for the treatment of African Americans with congestive heart failure, viewing it as a sign that the biomedical community and the U.S. government were finally taking seriously the health of this population and the responsibility of these parties to address what was seen largely as a product of their past neglect. These actions were also seen as a sign of movement toward true inclusion in the research and funding for chronic, life-threatening ailments. As Pollock questions, however, what good is inclusion at this point in the biomedical process when so many individuals for whom the drug was indicated either lacked the resources to obtain medical care in the first place, or were unable to pay for the drugs once they were prescribed? Regardless of whether BiDil is in fact a "Black drug," its failure to deliver projected profits reveals that even the best drugs only work if they can actually be delivered to their intended recipients. Nadine Ehlers and Shiloh Krupar address the risks of inclusion by the example of targeting operations (medical hot spotting) that direct health care to particular populations in particular spaces. They show that despite the fact that medical hot spotting seeks to include minorities in the fold of health care, the practices' very logic is structured through an enduring epistemology of anti-Blackness. This form of "inclusion," as their account shows, actually represents a new modality of racialized administration, one that paradoxically augments Black exclusion from the general population. Catherine Bliss discusses the ways research inclusion by race became the predominant biomedical solution to solving racial inequality. Genomic inclusion was framed as the best redress for historical government neglect of minority communities. In focusing on genomic research, however, economic and political understandings of race and health were sidelined. Without a simultaneous focus on these other factors affecting the health of minority communities, genomic solutions to eradicating health disparities are doomed in advance to failure. On a related point, Ruha Benjamin and Leslie Hinkson argue that the original aim of inclusion as a means of historical redress has been diluted through reframing it in the language of diversity. While not central to their arguments, both Bliss's and Benjamin and Hinkson's chapters note that as the language around inclusion shifted gears, the prospective beneficiaries of inclusion changed as well. In biomedicine, this portends an increase in minority participants in clinical trials and also in organ and tissue sample donation that may, at the end of the day, serve to provide benefits primarily to nonminority individuals and to biomedicine itself, at least in part because of the lack of access to health services that disproportionately affects minority communities.

How can inclusion be reimagined to actually begin operating as a form of reparative justice? Reparation might be achieved in the first instance by ensuring that minority and low-income individuals actually have access to the care and services that the results of their inclusion in the research process have made possible. Access here would mean not simply the capacity to acquire adequate health insurance but also the ability to obtain affordable, quality care. In a second sense, inclusion might also function as a form of reparative justice via the research design phase: when recruiting minority subjects, more attention could be paid to how they specifically will benefit from the results of their inclusion. While the supposed genetic diversity their participation will provide to the research endeavor more broadly is indeed a significant reason to ensure their inclusion, experiments and trials surely must also be designed with an eye toward targeting the health problems that disproportionately affect minority communities—but, again, in ways that avoid essentializing race. In this way, inclusion can simultaneously further the diversity aims of the biomedical research apparatus and at least have greater potential to fulfill the original aim of setting right health disparities that are in large part due to a series of historical medical and societal wrongs. In a third sense, in the pursuit of greater inclusion of minorities in biomedical research, reparations might be made by giving greater respect and attention to the lived experience of minorities in this society. Without the proper attention paid to the environmental, economic, and social conditions within which minorities live (and in many cases in which they were raised), race turns into a variable that has little power to help inform us about existing health disparities, how to ameliorate them today, and how to eradicate them in the future. Unless we are careful in thinking through how we design our research, how we approach analysis, and how we interpret our findings as they relate to race, merely increasing the number of minorities in the research phase will prove to be of little benefit to the communities these studies are thought to represent.

The United States is today in a cultural moment that demands not just a heightened focus on racial inequality but also sustained critique of how race itself is understood and continues to matter across multiple areas in American society. For example, in examining the criminal justice system, a growing number of the American public, and at a slower pace its public officials, have begun to question policing practices that disproportionately target, punish, and endanger Black and Brown individuals in the name of law and order. In another example, in higher education, more and more minority youth and their allies are questioning the commitment to diversity held by colleges and universities that seemingly do very little to dispel the notions that minority students are the only ones who benefit under diversity policies, that all minority students are beneficiaries of this policy, and that minority students, along with their coursework, their extracurriculars, and sometimes jobs and unpaid internships, are somehow also responsible for providing a diverse experience for their classmates. They are also pushing educational institutions on issues of reparative justice—how much does this institution owe to the prior institutions of slavery and indentured servitude?—and on the lauding of individuals whose names appear on buildings and statues who overtly and unapologetically contributed to the oppression of minority groups. In a final example, the boycott of the 2016 Oscars, while seemingly trivial, sheds light on the lack of diversity in the representation of minorities in the media. More importantly, this boycott pushes us to question why so few minorities are in positions of creative authority in cultural fields, especially film; why so few executives understand that the stories of racial minorities have broad global appeal and the potential to yield profits; and why there are so few minorities in the visual field.

These are just a few of the struggles and movements that are building momentum in the United States as of this writing. They all push us to question whether in America today "all men are created equal" and the extent to which one's racial categorization either ensures or undermines one's claim to equality. While there is both a movement to increase access to health care for minority populations and to decrease perceived discrimination in the quality of care minority patients receive, there is very little push for questioning the content of biomedical knowledge, the aims of the biomedical research community, or the dispersion of benefits accrued from biomedical research as it relates to race. This is a moment for those committed to social medicine and sound medical practice to begin challenging medical practitioners and researchers on their insistence of using race as either a biological reality or a good-enough proxy for biological "truth" in the absence of confirmed scientific evidence. In no other movement noted above are the activists pushing against an articulation of race as biological fact or innate, hardwired cultural deficiency. In some ways, that would make their struggles easier. After all, so many Americans seem to be aware at least of the idea of race as a social construction. The extent to which they understand this is, of course, debatable. If police officers and prosecutors asserted explicitly that the disproportionate number of minorities fined, prosecuted, imprisoned, surveilled, and injured or killed by the police and the courts was due to some innate biological or cultural difference, how much greater would the outcry we are witnessing today be? What if colleges and universities issued a broad public statement that censured minority protest over admissions policies and the racial climate of these institutions with an argument based on purported biologically based intellectual deficiencies of minorities who should simply be grateful for being allowed into these rarified spaces in the first place? What if Hollywood, in its defense of failing to support minority filmmakers and writers, and its unwillingness to invest in minority-made projects, went with a rationale of race-based deficiencies in creativity, plot complexity, or imagination as opposed to its old line on lack of marketability, both at home and globally? These arguments would be seen as unsavory, as constitutionally untenable, and as racist, and thus as incompatible with American values. How is it, then, that this logic is able to go so comparatively uncontested in race-based medicine?

We hope that this volume inspires those who read it to not only question the biological reality of race but to act against its use in biomedicine. The contributors to this volume are representative of fields across the humanities and social sciences in which there are real proscriptions against setting forth normative claims in scholarly work. Even given that, throughout this volume we have, in some cases more explicitly than others, stated our rejection of the use of race as biological reality in medical research and practice in both empirical and ethical terms. The use of race in biomedicine should not be viewed as sacrosanct because the level of expertise of those who are involved in the field is perceived as being so much more specialized and empirically grounded than those of us in the social sciences and humanities and even in the lay public. Biomedical knowledge and assumptions, as in other fields, are culturally informed. If we as a culture collectively push against biologized notions of race across all fields, including biomedicine, we can begin a revolution of thought and practice that would actualize an alternative racial future.

Notes

1. On "racial project," see Michael Omi and Howard Winant, *Racial Formation in the United States: From the 1960s to the 1990s* (New York: Routledge, 2014).

2. John P. Geyman, "Myths as Barriers to Health Care Reform in the United States," *International Journal of Health Services* 33, no. 2 (2003): 315–29.

3. For further investigation of such a possibility, see Jonathan M. Metzl and Helena Hansen, "Structural Competency: Theorizing a New Medical Engagement with Stigma and Inequality," *Social Science and Medicine* 103 (2014): 126–33.

4. Richard Herrnstein and Charles Murray, *The Bell Curve: Intelligence and Class Structure in American Life* (New York: Simon & Shuster, 1994).

5. See, for example, Lundy Braun, "Race, Ethnicity, and Health: Can Genetics Explain Disparities?," *Perspectives in Biology and Medicine* 45, no. 2 (2002): 159–74; "Style Matters: Describing Race, Ethnicity, and Culture in Medical Research," *British Medical Journal* 312, no. 7038 (1996): 1054–55; Richard S. Cooper, Jay S. Kaufman, and Ryk Ward, "Race and Genomics," *New England Journal of Medicine* 348, no. 12 (2003): 1166–70; Mindy Thompson Fullilove, "Comment: Abandoning 'Race' as a Variable in Public Health Research—An Idea Whose Time Has Come," *American Journal of Public Health* 88, no. 9 (1998): 1297–98; Judith B. Kaplan and Trude Bennett, "Use of Race and Ethnicity in Biomedical Publication," *JAMA*, 289 no. 20 (2003): 2709–16; Newton G. Osborne and Marvin D. Feit, "The Use of Race in Medical Research," *JAMA*, 267, no. 2 (1992): 275–79; Elizabeth G. Phimister, "Medicine and the Racial Divide," *New England Journal of Medicine,* 348, no. 12 (2003): 1081–82; Robert S. Schwartz, "Racial Profiling in Medical Research," editorial, *New England Journal of Medicine* 344, no.18 (2001): 1392–93; Ritchie Witzig, "The Medicalization of Race: Scientific Legitimization of a Flawed Social Construct," *Annals of Internal Medicine* 125, no. 8 (1996): 675–79.

ACKNOWLEDGMENTS

The idea for this book germinated several years ago, when the editors responded to a call for panels for the American Studies Association annual meeting. The theme of that conference, held in Washington, D.C., in 2013, was "Beyond the Logic of Debt, Toward an Ethics of Collective Dissent." The meeting invited participants to explore the dominant logics of debt in practical, material, and institutional contexts. Such a call encouraged us to think about the work we had been doing independently on race-based medicine through the lens of debt—which, as we were to find, yielded an incredibly rich forum for analysis. We would like to thank the Program Committee of the 2013 ASA for the impetus to extend the concept of debt to racialized medicine. We would also like to thank the Committee of Ethnic Studies of the American Studies Association for sponsoring the panel, and Ricardo Ortiz (chair, Department of English, Georgetown University, and at the time the chair of the Standing Committee of Ethnic Studies of the ASA) for his support of both the panel and the idea behind it. This initial recognition of the salience of our focus eventually led us to conceive the panel topic as an edited volume. Developing the panel papers and topic into a book would not have been possible, however, without our contributors—Ruha Benjamin, Catherine Bliss, Khiara Bridges, Shiloh Krupar, Jenna Loyd, and Anne Pollock. While some of these authors were part of the initial panel, others joined us along the way. We thank each of them for their participation in this venture and for their insightful analyses that enrich our understandings of the stakes of race-based medicine.

Jason Weidemann welcomed this book at the University of Minnesota Press, and we thank him for his support and his conviction about the importance of this topic. We could not have asked for a better editor or for a more seamless progression from concept to completion. Thanks also to Erin Warholm-Wohlenhaus, who guided the book through production. Our anonymous reviewers provided valuable suggestions that helped crystallize our thinking, and the book is richer because of their attention. We are grateful to them for their sustained engagement with the individual chapters and the intellectual generosity with which they approached the project as a whole.

Nadine Ehlers would like to thank her coeditor, Leslie Hinkson, for embarking on this project and for being an incredible collaborator and advocate. She would also like to extend gratitude to her coauthor and interlocutor, Shiloh Krupar, along with Clare Armitage, Donette Francis, Arabella Hayes, and Kirsty Nowlan, for their ongoing sustenance. She thanks her family for being family and Taariq Lewis for the questions and the journey.

Leslie Hinkson, not to be a copycat, would also like to thank her coeditor, Nadine Ehlers, not just for her work as collaborator and her friendship but also for being a phenomenal mentor. She would also like to thank her coauthor, Ruha Benjamin, for allowing her to hitch her wagon to what was already an excellent project on its own. Thanks should also be extended to Debbie Becher, Cristina Mora, and Anna Zajacova for their support in developing and critiquing her earliest work on race-based medicine and on keeping her sane and grounded on the road toward tenure. Finally, she would like to thank her family, Matthew, Olivia, Althea, and Una. Without them, she would be measuring out her life with coffee spoons instead of simply and happily living it.

CONTRIBUTORS

RUHA BENJAMIN is assistant professor of African American studies at Princeton University and faculty affiliate for the Program on History of Science, Center for Health and Wellbeing, Program on Gender and Sexuality, Program in Global Health and Health Policy, and Department of Sociology. She is a research associate in the Centre for Indian Studies in Africa at the University of Witwatersrand and author of *People's Science: Bodies and Rights on the Stem Cell Frontier*.

CATHERINE BLISS is assistant professor of sociology at the University of California, San Francisco. Her research explores the sociology of race, gender, and sexuality in science and society. Her book *Race Decoded: The Genomic Fight for Social Justice* examines how genomics became today's new science of race. Her latest project examines convergences in social and genetic science in the postgenomic age, including implications for equality, identity, and belonging.

KHIARA M. BRIDGES is professor of law and anthropology at Boston University. She has written many articles concerning race, class, reproductive rights, and the intersection of the three. Her scholarship has been published in the *Stanford Law Review*, the *Columbia Law Review*, and the *California Law Review*, among others. She is author of *Reproducing Race: An Ethnography of Pregnancy as a Site of Racialization* and *The Poverty of Privacy Rights*.

NADINE EHLERS joined the Department of Sociology and Social Policy at the University of Sydney in 2016. Previously she held appointments at Georgetown University, the University of North Carolina, Greensboro,

The Ohio State University, and the University of Wollongong. Her research centers on the sociocultural study of the body, law, and biomedicine to examine the racial and gendered governance of individuals and populations. She is author of *Racial Imperatives: Discipline, Performativity, and Struggles against Subjection.*

LESLIE R. HINKSON is assistant professor of sociology at Georgetown University. Her research explores the role and meaning of race across institutional contexts and its effects on educational, employment, and health outcomes. She had a postdoctoral fellowship with the Robert Wood Johnson Health Policy Research Fellows at the University of Michigan and is completing a monograph, *The Limits to School Integration: Lessons on American Racism from Department of Defense Schools.*

SHILOH KRUPAR is a geographer, Provost's Distinguished associate professor, and field chair of the culture and politics program in the Walsh School of Foreign Service at Georgetown University. Her teaching and research interests span geography, architecture, museum studies, medical humanities, and environmental justice. She is author of *Hot Spotter's Report: Military Fables of Toxic Waste* (Minnesota, 2013) and serves as interim codirector of the National Toxic Land/Labor Conservation Service (with Sarah Kanouse, Northeastern University).

JENNA M. LOYD is assistant professor in the Zilber School of Public Health and a member of the urban studies program faculty at University of Wisconsin–Milwaukee. She is author of *Health Rights Are Civil Rights: Peace and Justice Activism in Los Angeles, 1963–1978* (Minnesota, 2014). She is coeditor, with Matt Mitchelson and Andrew Burridge, of *Beyond Walls and Cages: Prisons, Borders, and Global Crisis,* which received the Past President Book Gold Award from the Association of Borderland Studies.

ANNE POLLOCK is associate professor of science, technology, and society in the School of Literature, Media, and Communication at Georgia Tech. She is author of *Medicating Race: Heart Disease and Durable Preoccupations with Difference.* She continues to research race and medicine in the United States while writing her second book, which is based on ethnographic research in South Africa.

INDEX

access to healthcare, racial inequality in, vii–ix, 62–66, 190–94
ACE inhibitors, race and gender differences in use of, 14–19
Adarand Constructors, Inc. v. Peña, 155
admissions procedures: constitutional color-blindness and, 159–61, 192–94; equal protection jurisprudence and, 175–77; individuation versus deindividuation debate over, 168–72, 180n45; metaphysics of, 162–67, 180n45
affirmative action, 155–57; admissions metaphysics and, 162–67, 182n53; ethnopharmacogenomics and, 157–61; race-based medicine and, xxiii–xxiv, 175–77
Affordable Care Act: political negotiations for, 70–71; race-based medicine and, xxii, 57–58, 186–87, xxviin19; racial disparities in insurance and, 90–92; racial politics surrounding, 59–62; Republican defunding of, 56–58; sovereign debt and, 55–75; temporality, value, and death in debate over, 62–66

African-American Heart Failure Trial (A-HeFT), 85
African Americans: BiDil heart failure medication targeted to, 83–101, 113–16; distrust of medicine by, 129–33, 138–40, 147–48, 151n29; drug trial recruitment of, xxiii, 85–101, 113–16, 132–33; gene-environment research on, 121–23; healthcare inequality for, xi–xxv; medical hot spotting of, 39–44; science and medicine and, 131–33; stagnation of middle class growth for, viii
African Genome Diversity Project, 114–16, 118–20
agency, slow death and, 62–66
Aid to Families with Dependent Children (AFDC), 68–69
American College of Surgeons, 67
American Hospital Association, 70–71
American Medical Association (AMA), 67, 68
anti-Blackness: defined, 47n8; medical hot spotting and, 41–44, 51n54; race-based biomedical targeting and, 34

antihypertensive medications, race and gender differences in use of, 14–15
Asian Americans, race and science and, 131–33
Asia Pacific Economic Cooperation Summit, 59
Association of Black Cardiologists (ABC), 89, 113
"attrition of the subject," health status and, 62–66
Axelrod, David, 70–71

Bell, Joyce M., 137–38
Bell Curve, The (Herrnstein and Murray), 189
benevolence, in race-based medicine, xx
Benjamin, Ruha, xxiii, 129–47, 187, 191
Berlant, Lauren, 62–66, 73–74
Bernanke, Ben, 58
beta-blockers, 185; color-blind racialized use of, 20–21; race and gender differences in use of, 14–19
Bhabha, Homi, 145
BiDil heart failure medication, xvii, 5, 35–36, 47n7, 187; compensation relations and politics of, 83, 93–101; development of, 85–92, 190–91; race-specific clinical trials for, 113–16
binaries: biomedicine and, 136–37; group-based racial classification and, 172–75
bioconstitutionalism: color-blindness and, 155–61; stem cell research and, 135–37
biological citizenship: medical hot spotting and, 41, 50n37; stem cell research and, 135–37
biological determinism, race and science and, 131–33
biomedicine: binaries and, 136–37; color-blind policies and, 109–12, 157–61; debt and, 186–94; ethnopharmacogenomics and, 169–72; ethnoracial classifications in, 129; individuation in, 179n19; profit orientation in, 4–5; race-specific biomedical targeting, 33–36, 112–16; racial segmentation in, xiii–xiv, xxiv–xxv, 9, 23–24; reparations and redemption and, 131–33; research funding for, 188–94; sociology of race and, 116–20; trust of institutions in, 138–40
biopolitics of health: disposability and, xii, 48n11; medical hot spotting and, 41–44; minstrelsy and charismatic collaborations and, 143–47; race-specific biomedical targeting, 33–36, 183–94; sovereign indebtedness discourse and, 57–58. *See also* race-based medicine
Birgeneau, Robert, 137
birther conspiracy theory, 61–62
bivariate statistical analysis, racial patterns in hypertension management and, 12
Black Lives Matter movement, 45–46
Black women: pharmaceutical prescriptions for, xxi–xxii; subprime lending targeting, 7–8
Bliss, Catherine, 107–24, 188–89, 191
Boehner, John, 56
Bratton, William, 42–44
Brenner, Jeffrey, 36–39, 42–44, 49n24
Brewster, Lizzy M., 21
Bridges, Khiara M., xxiii, 155–77, 189–90
Broad Institute, 117–18
Brown, Michael, 63
Bush, George W., 66, 69–70
Bush, Haydn, 31
Byrd, W. Michael, 61–62, 65

calcium channel blockers (CCBs), race and gender differences in use of, 14–19
California Institute for Regenerative Medicine, 133–40, 144–47
California Stem Cell Act, 136
Callon, Michel, 144
Camden Coalition of Healthcare Providers, 36–39
Camden Healthcare Providers Breakfast Group, 36–39
Cantor, Eric, 56
capitalism: healthcare reform and role of, 66–71; slow death and, 62–66; whiteness and accumulation of, 71–74
Carbado, Devon W., 164–65
Center for Research on Genomics and Global Health, 119, 121
Centers for Disease Control and Prevention: Office of Public Health Genomics, 121; research on race and public health by, 110
Centers for Population Health and Health Disparities, 120
Centers of Excellence in Ethical, Social, and Legal Issues Research, 120–21
Centre d'Etude du Polymorphisme Humain, 109
charismatic collaboration, biopolitics and, 143–47
Children's Health Insurance Plan (CHIP), 69–71
class: health care reform and, 66–71; individuation and, 171–72
Clayton, Linda A., 61–62, 65
clinical gatekeepers, research and, 140–46
Clinton, Bill, healthcare reform and, 69
Clinton, Hillary, 55
CNN Money, 58

Cohn, Jay, 113–14
color-blind policies: Affordable Care Act politics and, 60–62; biomedical targeting and, 35–36; ethnopharmacogenomics and, 157–61; in genomics research, 109–12; racial inequality in healthcare and, xiii–xiv; racialization of medications and, 19–21; scientific research and, 116–20; Supreme Court rulings and, 155–57, 177n2, 178n8
Common Fund (NIH), 122
community outreach, drug marketing through, 86–92
compensation relations, BiDil heart failure medication and role of, 83, 93–101
CompStat, 37–39
Congressional Black Caucus, 86
constitutional color-blindness, equal protection jurisprudence and, 155–61
copays for drugs, 89–92
costs of healthcare: conditions of lethality and, 39–44; economic policies and, 22–24; freedom from debt and, 183–94; gender disparities in, 17–19; medical errors and, 8–9; medical hot spotting and, 36–39; Medicare and Medicaid passage and increase in, 68; racial disparities in, 8, 13, 15–19, 21–22; uncompensated care debt, 32; U.S. economic competitiveness and, 70–71
creditors, race-based medicine and, xx
crime mapping, medical hot spotting compared with, 42–44
Cruz, Ted, 58, 59
cultural issues: distrust of research and, 139–40; race-based medicine and, xxiii, 189–94

cystic fibrosis, race-based medicine and, 22

Daly, Mark, 117–18
Davis, Chantel, 63
Davis, Mike, 73
debt: BiDil heart failure medication and role of, 83–101; compensation relations and, 93–101; defined, xv; freedom from, 183–94; health care inequality and, x–xxv; health policy framing with, 63–66; housing bubble and aggravation of, 3–4; medical hot spotting and, 39–44; race-based medicine and, ix–xxv, 183–94. *See also* uncompensated care debt
debtors, race-based medicine and, xx
deficit reduction, debt ceiling and, 58–62
deindividuation, race and, 168–69
Department of Energy, genome research and, 111–12, 120
Department of Health and Human Services (HHS): gene-environment research and, 120, 122; genomics research and, 110–16, 120; racial disparities in healthcare access and, x, xxvin11, 65–66, 110
dependency, race-based medicine and, xxii–xxiii
Derickson, Alan, 67
Derrida, Jacques, 131
Dillon, Michael, 33
Directive No. 15 (OMB), 110–12, 114; biology of race and, 116–20
direct-to-consumer advertising, BiDil case and use of, 88–92
disintegration of bodies: healthcare reform and, 67–71; wealth gap and, 62–66
disparities in healthcare: freedom from debt and, 184–94; gender and, 17–19, 66–71; gene-environment research and, 116–20; Human Genome Project and, 109–12; meaning of, 107–24; racial differences in communication and, 130; racial disparities, 8, 13, 15–19, 21–22
diuretics: color-blind racialization of, 20–21; race and gender differences in use of, 14–19
diversity rationale: constitutional color-blindness and, 159–61; equal protection jurisprudence and, 175–77, 192–94; individuation versus deindividuation debate and, 168–69; racial profiling versus, 137–40
drug development, race-based medicine and, xiv, xviii, 5
drug trial recruitment: biopolitical minstrelsy and, 143–47; clinical gatekeepers and subversive whiteness and, 140–46; racial patterns in, xxiii, 85–101, 113–16, 129–30, 132–33, 137–40, 147–48, 151n29
Du Bois, W. E. B., xi, 33, 34, 64
Dunston, Georgia, 114, 118–19
Duster, Troy, xix, 116–18, 123–24

earnings patterns, racial inequality in, viii
economic policies: health care access and, 50n38, 107–9; race-based medicine and, 22–24
efficacy studies, race-based differences in hypertension treatment and, 17–19
eligibility-based models, admissions procedures and, 162–67
Emanuel, Rahm, 70–71
emergency medicine: African American use of, xxvin11; medical hot spotting, 37–39

INDEX   205

employer-based health insurance, decline of, 67–71
employment rates, racial inequality in, viii
end-of-life care, racial differences in communication during, 130
epigenomics, race in context of, 116–20
Epstein, Steven, 132, 144
equal protection jurisprudence: affirmative action and, 155–57, 159–61, 182n53; color-blind policies and, 155–57; ethnopharmacogenomics and, 157–61; group identity and individuation under, 172–75; individuation versus deindividuation and, 168–69; injury of racial classifications and, 168; race-based medicine and, 169–72, 175–77
Espeland, Michael, 166–67
Espeland, Wendy, 166–67
ethics: of medical hot spotting, 44–46; race-based medicine and, 115–16
ethnopharmacogenomics, xiv, xviii; color-blind policies and, 157–61; defined, 161–62; evolution of, 113–16; group identity and, 172–75; health disparities and, 107–9; individuation and, 158–61, 169–72, 179n21; profit motivation in, 5
excess death, Du Bois's concept of, 64–66

federal debt ceiling, Affordable Care Act defunding and, 56–62
Federalist Papers, 57
Fisher v. Texas II, 175
Food and Drug Administration: BiDil approval, 85; race-specific pharmaceuticals and, xxii; race-specific pharmacokinetics and pharmacodynamics mandate, 112–16
foreign policy, sovereign debt politics and, 59–62
formularies, drug status in, 91–92
Foucault, Michel, 33
Fox, Michael J., 143
FreedomWorks, 56–58
Fryer, Roland, 20

Gaskin, Richard, 143–47, 153n50, 153n53
Gates, Henry Louis, Jr., 20
Geiger, H. Jack, 59–60, 66, 79n63
gender: differences antihypertensive medications based on, 14–19; genomics research and, 111–12; health disparities and, 66–71; identity politics and, 55–56; mortality rates and, 65–66; race-based medical decision making and, 16–19
Gene-Environment Initiative, 122
gene-environment research: race in context of, 116–20; reparations and, 120–23
Genehunter program, 117–18
generic equivalents, unbranding of drugs and, 92
genomics: evolution of, 109–12; race-based medicine and, 112–16, 184–94; race in context of, xxxn43, 107–9, 116–20, 123–24. *See also* ethnopharmacogenomics
geodemographics, medical hot spotting and, 42–44
Geographic Information Systems (GIS), medical hot spotting and, 31, 42–44
Geronimus, Arline, 65–66
Gilmore, Ruth Wilson, 64, 73–74
Ginsberg, Ruth Bader, 63
Giroux, Henry, xii, 36, 48n11

Global Health Initiative, 122
Global South, race-based medicine in, 115–16
Goldberg, David Theo, 60
Goldstein, Alyosha, xv–xvi
Good, Mary-Jo DelVecchio, 146
Gordon, Avery, 62, 64–66, 73–74
government shutdown, Affordable Care Act funding and, 58–62
government spending, race-based medicine and, xx
graduate institutions, admissions procedures in, 165–67
Grant, Oscar, 63
Great Recession, socioeconomic impact of, 3–4
group identity: ethnopharmacogenomics and, 158–62; individuation and, 172–75
Grutter v. Bollinger, 159, 175–76

Happe, Kelly, xix–xx
Harris, Cheryl I., 146, 164–65
Hartman, Saidiya, xvi, 137–38
Hartmann, Douglas, 137–38
haunting, in Affordable Care Act debate, 64–66, 73–74
Haynes, M. Alfred, 64–65
hazardous site exposure, racial inequality in healthcare and, xiii
Head Start program, 57
health care system: class and racial exclusion in, 66–71; racial inequality in access to, viii–ix, 62–66; wealth inequality and, x–xxv
health insurance: access to, 89–92; early proposals for, 67–68
Health People 2000, 65
health status, politics of, 62–66
Healthy People statement, 110
hegemonic whiteness, race-based medicine and, 141

Herrnstein, Richard, 189
Hill-Burton Act, 67
Hoffman, Sharona, xvii
homicide deaths, declines in, 65–66
hospitals: African American use of, xxvin11, xxixn37; federal funding for construction of, 67–68; racial inequality in access to, xvi–xvii
Hossler, Don, 162
House Freedom Caucus, 75
housing market, racial profiling and valuation in, 6–8
Howard University, 114, 118
Hughey, Matthew, 141
human body: ethnopharmacogenomics and, 159–61; individuation of race and, 169–72
Human Genome Diversity Project, 111–12
Human Genome Project, 109–12, 114
Human Health and Heredity in Africa Project, 119–20
hydrochlorothiazides, racialized use of, 20–21
hypertension: race and gender differences in treatment of, 14–15, 24; race-based treatment of, 10–13, 14–19

identity politics, race and gender and, 55–56
"I Have a Dream" speech (King), 156
inclusion and difference paradigm, racial distrust of science and medicine and, 132–33, 190–94
indebtedness. *See* debt; monetary debt; uncompensated care debt
individual particularity: ethnopharmacogenomics and, 158–61, 169–72, 179n19, 179n21; group identity and, 172–75; race and, 168–69

INDEX

Inside Washington, 58
institutionalization of health research, gene-environment research, 120–23
insured status, lower rates for African Americans and minorities, x, xxviin19
International HapMap Project, 114–16, 119
interventions in health care: Black–White difference in response to, 20–21; medical hot spotting and, 42–44
IQ scores, racial assumptions concerning, 189

James, Angela, xxxn45
Jasanoff, Sheila, 135
Johnson, John M., 129
Johnson, Lyndon, 68
Joint National Committee on Detection, Evaluation, and Treatment of High Blood Pressure (JNC) reports, 10–19
justifiable homicides, statistics on, 63–66, 78n42

Kalsbeek, David, 162
Kennedy, John F., 68
Kennedy, Ted, 143
Kerr–Mills Eldercare plan, 68
King, Dr. Martin Luther, Jr., vii, 156
Krauthammer, Charles, 55–56, 58, 64, 73
Krupar, Shiloh, xxi–xxii, 31–46, 186, 191

Lander, Eric, 114
Laurent, Louise, 139
Law School Admissions Council (LSAC), 165–67
Law School Admission Test (LSAT), 166–67, 181n50

lethality, medical hot spotting and, 39–44
letters of recommendation, admissions procedures and, 165
Limbaugh, Rush, 61, 64, 72
Lizza, Ryan, 59–60
Lott, Eric, 145
Loyd, Jenna M., xxii, 55–75, 186

Madison, James, 57
Mangano, Joseph, 65
marketing: BiDil heart failure medication and role of, 83–92; race-specific pharmaceuticals, xxii
Martin, Trayvon, 63
McCollum, Bill, 71
Meadows, Mark, 56, 58, 62, 75
Medicaid: cuts to, 68–69; entitlement paradox of, 69–71; exchanges, Affordable Care Act politics and, 59–62, 70–71; passage of, 68; unequal access to, 66–71
Medical Advisory Committee, 67
medical die-ins, 45–46
medical error, race-based decision-making and, 8–9
medical hot spotting: ethics of, 44–46, 191–94; evolution of, 31–32, 36–39, 48n19; growth of, 38–39; lethality conditions and, 39–44; militarized visual culture and, 53n68
Medicare, passage of, 68
medication, race and gender differences in use of, 14–19
Melamed, Jodi, 71–74
Melnikov, Andrew, 129
middle class, stagnation of African Americans in, viii
Miller v. Johnson, 160–61
monetary debt: BiDil heart failure medication and role of, 83–101;

freedom from, 183–94; race-based medicine and, xxi–xxii
moral debt: freedom from, 183–94; medicalization of structural racism and, 107–9; race-specific pharmaceuticals and, xxiii; racial distrust in stem cell science and, 129–47
morbidity rates, racial differences in, viii–ix, 65–66
mortality rates: class and racial exclusion and, 66–71; racial differences in, viii–ix, 64–66
mortgage default crisis, 3–4, 23–24
Mulvaney, Rick, 75
Murray, Charles, 189

NAACP, 86, 113
National Center for Health Statistics, 11–12
National Federation of Independent Businesses v. Sibelius, 59–63, 71
National Health and Nutrition Examination Survey (NHANES III), 12–13
National Healthcare Quality Report, x
National Heart, Lung, and Blood Institute (NHLBI), hypertension guidelines, 10
National Human Genome Research Center, 111–12, 114, 119–22
National Institute for Child Health and Human Development, 120
National Institutes of Health (NIH): Common Fund, 122; genomics research and, 110–12; health disparities research and, 120–23; Task Force on Obesity, 121–22
National Medical Association, 113
National Research Council, 111
Nature (magazine), 114

Neal, Andrew W., 33
neoliberalism: biomedical targeting and, 34–36; medical hot spotting and, 40–44; racial inequities in healthcare and, xi–xii; racial neoliberalism, 60–62
New England Journal of Medicine, 113
New York Times, 59
NIH Intramural Center for Health Disparities Genomics, 119
NIH Pharmacogenomics Research Network, 115
nitric oxide deficiency, 185
NitroMed, 86
Nixon, Richard, 68
normativity, diversity outreach versus racial profiling and, 137–40
Norris, Keith, 138–39
Nunes, Devin, 72–73

Obama, Barack, 59, 122; racial politics and presidency of, 55–56, 61
obesity crisis: gene-environment research and, 121–22; politics of agency and, 62–66
Oliver, Melvin L., vii
Omnibus Budget Reconciliation Acts, 68–69
Oregon Health Insurance Experiment, 66
O'Reilly, Bill, 61–62
Orientalist anxiety, health care politics and, 73–74

Palin, Sarah, 81n86
Pallavicini, Maria, 138–40
Parents Involved in Community Schools v. Seattle School District No. 1, xiii
patient-focused accountable care,

medical hot spotting and, 44–46, 50n37
patient noncompliance, racial patterns in, 141
Patient Protection and Affordable Care Act. *See* Affordable Care Act
Pemberton, Stephen, 142–43
performance-based models, admissions procedures and, 162–67
personalized medicine, genomics and, 107–9
personal responsibility paradigm: medical hot spotting and, 42–44, 52n58; racial inequities in healthcare and, xi–xii
personal statement, in admissions procedures, 168–72, 180n45
pharmaceutical industry: BiDil case study and, 85–101, 102n12; race-based medicine and, xiv, xxi–xxiii, 47n7
pharmacogenomics, 161–62; advances in, 180n30
Pharmacogenomics Journal, 113
pharmacokinetics and pharmacodynamics, race-specific analysis of, 112–16
pharmakon metaphor, 131
Philadelphia Negro, The (Du Bois), xi
physicians: drug marketing focus on, 86–92, 102n12; nonverbal communication by, racial differences in, 130
Planned Parenthood, 75
police violence: racial profiling and, 192–94; slow death of uninsured compared with, 63–66, 78n42
political geography, race and, 59–62
politics, medical hot spotting and, 42–44

Pollock, Anne, xxii, 19–20, 83–101, 131, 187
Ponder, C. S., 6–7
population demographics: genomics research and, 110–12; medical hot spotting and, 36–39
power dynamics: BiDil heart failure medication and role of, 83–101; healthcare inequality and, xii
predatory lending practices, 3–4
premature deaths, healthcare debate and, 64–66, 73–74
prescription drugs: racialized patterns in treatment involving, 5–6, 14–19; racial patterns in use of, xxviiin36; targeting of Black women, xxi–xxii. *See also specific drug genres*
private insurance, union support for, 67
privatized health care, racial inequities and, xi–xii
Proposition 71 (California), 133–37
public health: color-blind policies in, 109–12; genomics and, 107–9, 121–23; race-based medicine and, xxii, 123–24
Publicis, 86

race: definitions of, xviii–xxv; genomics research and classifications of, 110–12; healthcare politics and, 59–62; identity politics and, 55–56; individuating versus de-individuating debate over, 168–69; in scientific context, 116–20
race-based medicine: BiDil heart failure medication and, 83–101, 114–16; biomedical targeting, 33–35; categories of, xx; clinical gatekeepers and subversive whiteness and, 140–46; color-blind

drugs, racialization of, 19–21; cost disparities in treatment and, 13, 15–19; debt burden and, ix–xvii; decision making in, 6–8; definitions of, xvii–xxv, xxxn45; discourse over, ix; economic access to care and, 50n38; equal protection jurisprudence and, 169–72, 175–77; ethnopharmacogenomics and, 157–61; ethnoracial classifications in, 129; genomics and, 107–9, 112–16, 118–20; health disparities and, 107–24; hypertension and, 10–13; individuation and, 169–72, 179n19; injury of racial classifications, 168; medical errors and, 8–9; profit orientation in, 4–5; redress and reparations and, 184–94; sovereign debt and, 57–75; stem cell research and, 133–37
race-specific biobank proposal, 115–16
race-targeted medical hot spotting, xxi–xxii
racial inequality: bodily harm of, 64–66; color-blind policies and, 155–57; continuing problem of, vii–xxv; health care reform and, 66–71; health disparities and, 8, 13, 15–19, 21–22, 107–24; impact of Great Recession on, 3–4; predatory lending and, 3–4; race-based medicine and, xviii
racial neoliberalism, 60–62
racial profiling: of BiDil heart failure medication, 83–101; decision making in race-based medicine and, 6–8; ethnopharmacogenomics and, 161–62; in health system use analysis, xxi–xxii; medical errors and, 8–9; trial recruitment and, 137–40

racial valuation: Affordable Care Act politics and, 56–62; decision making in race-based medicine and, 6–9
racism: definition of, 64; genomic health effects of, 115–16; stem cell science, moral debt and, 129–47
Randolph, A. Philip, 68
rankings systems, admissions procedures and, 166
Ratigan, Dylan, 31
rationing of medical care, 81n86; racialized patterns of, 7–8
Reagan, Ronald, 68–69
Reardon, Jenny, 146
redress and reparations: Affordable Care Act characterized as, 71–74; equal protection jurisprudence and, 175–77; freedom from debt and, 183–94; gene-environment research and, 120–24; genomics and, 107–9, 114–15, 123–24; slave health deficit and, 61–62; stem cell research and, 135–37
Reeve, Christopher, 143–44
Reeve, Dana, 143
Regents of the University of California v. Bakke, 182n53
Republican Party: sovereign debt and Affordable Care Act politics and, 56–58; suicide caucus of, 57–62
research: funding proposals for, 188–94; racial patterns in distrust of, 129–33, 138–40, 147–48, 151n29
Revitalization Act of 1993, 110
right to research, stem cell initiative and, 133–37
Risch, Neil, 115
Roberts, Dorothy, xvii, 55, 57, 178n8
Roberts, John (Chief Justice), xiii, 71
Romney, Mitt, 60

Roosevelt, Franklin Delano, 67
Rotimi, Charles, 114, 119, 121
Ruaño, Gualberto, 113
Ryan, Paul, 75

salt-slavery hypothesis, race-based medicine and, 20–21
Scalia, Antonin (Justice), 156–57
Scarborough, Joe, 60–61
schizophrenia, racially-based diagnoses of, xiii
scientific truth: in race-based medicine, xx; race in terms of, 116–20
Scott-Heron, Gil, 74
Second Bill of Rights, 67
Seedat, Yackoob K., 21
Sehgal, Ashwini, 20
self-care, medical hot spotting and, 41–46, 50n37
self-determination, racial characterizations of, 75n3
self-interest, in race-based medicine, xx
sequestration, debt ceiling and, 58–62
Shapiro, Thomas M., vii
sickle cell disease: failed expectations concerning, 142–43, 153n48; race-based medicine and, 141; stem cell research and, 134–37, 141–42
16 Candles (film), 73
slave health deficit, 61–62
slavery, origins of healthcare inequality in, xi–xiii
slow death, capitalism, politics and agency and, 62–66, 73–74
Smith, David Barton, 67–68
Social Security Administration, 67
social wage, longevity and, 62–66
sociology of race: biomedicine and, 188–94; charismatic collaboration and biopolitical minstrelsy, 143–47; ethnopharmacogenomics and, 157–61; freedom from debt and, 184–94; genetics research and, 116–20, 122–24; health disparities and, 107–9; individuation and, 171–72; race-based medicine and, 190–91; science and medicine and, 131–33
Southern exceptionalism, ACA politics and, 59–62
sovereign debt: fiscal cliff politics and, 58–62; race-based medicine and, 56–58
spatial ontology: expectations and, 52n61; medical hot spotting and, 42–44
Special Supplemental Nutrition Program for Women, Infants, and Children, 57
standardized testing, admissions procedures and, 163–67
statistical discrimination, racial profiling as, 9
stem cell research: charismatic collaboration and biopolitical minstrelsy concerning, 143–47; diversity outreach versus racial profiling in, 137–40; methods and background in, 133–37; moral debt and racial distrust of, 129–33
Stem Cell Research and Cures Act, 133–37
Stevens, Rosemary A., xii
structural racism: biomedical targeting and, 34–35; ethnopharmacogenomics and, 157–61; federal healthcare funding and, 67–71; medical hot spotting and, 41–44; medicalization of, 107–9; universal health care and, 57–58, 74
student capacity models, admissions procedures and, 162–67
student capacity to contribute models,

admissions procedures and, 162–67
subprime lending practices, racial patterns in, 6–8, 23–24
suicide caucus: politics over ACA and, 58–62, 72–74; racial geography and, 60
Supreme Court (U.S.): affirmative action dismantling by, xxiii–xxiv, 155–57; color-blindness in rulings by, 155–57, 177n2, 178n8; equal protection jurisprudence and, 168; racial classification laws and, 155–57
Synthetic Cohort for the Analysis of Longitudinal Effects of Gene-Environment Interactions, 122

Taft, Robert, xi–xii
TallBear, Kim, 146
tax cuts, debt ceiling and, 58–62
Tea Party, 56–58, 60, 72–73, 75
Thompson, Frank, 69–70
Troubled Dream of Genetic Medicine, The (Wailoo and Pemberton), 142–43
Truman, Harry, 67
Trump, Donald J., 74–75
trust: charismatic collaborations and, 143–47; clinical gatekeepers and subversive whiteness and, 141–46; race-based medicine and absence of, 129–33, 147–48, 151n29; in research, issues involving, 138–40
Tuskegee Syphilis Study, xiii, 140

uncompensated care debt, 32; medical hot spotting and, 40–46
underinsured populations, privatized health care and, xii
Unequal Treatment (Institute of Medicine), 66

uninsured populations: Affordable Care Act and, 63–66, 70–71; drug marketing and, 90–92; privatized health care and, xii; slow death of, 63–66
United Kingdom, hypertension guidelines in, 11
univariate statistical analysis, racial patterns in hypertension management and, 12
universal health care, race-based medicine and, 57–58, 74
"Use of Race and Ethnicity in Public Health Surveillance" (CDC), 110
U.S. News & World Report, academic rankings, 166–67

value, BiDil heart failure medication and role of, 83–101
Vigilante marketing firm, 86
violence, Orientalist framing of, 73–74

Wacquant, Loïc, 51n54
Wailoo, Keith, 142–43
Walcott, Rinaldo, xii–xiii
war imagery, Affordable Care Act politics and, 72–74
wealth gap: gender disparities in costs of healthcare and, 18–19; health care inequality and, x–xxv; health insurance coverage and, 69–71; impact of Great Recession on, 3–4; medical hot spotting and, 32; racial inequality and, viii, xxvin11; slow death concept and, 62–66
web-based marketing, BiDil case and use of, 88–92, 102n16
welfare policies: costs of, 75n9; Medicaid and, 68–69; penal policies and, 51n54
Westley, Robert, xv
white-coat die-ins, 45–46

whiteness: binaries in biomedicine and, 136–37; clinical gatekeepers and, 140–46; equal protection jurisprudence and, 175–77; wealth and, 71–74
"Whiteness as Property" (Harris), 146
Wilderson, Frank B., 47n8
W. M. Keck Center for Collaborative Neuroscience, 144
women: mortality rates for, 65–66; race-based cost disparities in medications for, 17–19

work experience, admissions procedures and, 165
Wright, Tate, 141
Wyly, Elvin, 6–7

Yancey, Antoinette, 144–45
Young, Wise, 144, 153n53

zero copay coupon, 89–92
"zones of black death," xii–xiii